Boko Pascal AKABASSI

Baobab, Kpassa or the plant with medicinal dexterity

Boko Pascal AKABASSI

Baobab, Kpassa or the plant with medicinal dexterity

Allossekpínmánssín or the prospect of health for all

ScienciaScripts

Imprint

Cover image: www.ingimage.com

This book is a translation from the original published under ISBN 978-620-6-71144-5.

Publisher:
Sciencia Scripts
is a trademark of
Dodo Books Indian Ocean Ltd. and OmniScriptum S.R.L publishing group

120 High Road, East Finchley, London, N2 9ED, United Kingdom
Str. Armeneasca 28/1, office 1, Chisinau MD-2012, Republic of Moldova, Europe
Printed at: see last page
ISBN: 978-620-8-07806-5

Contents

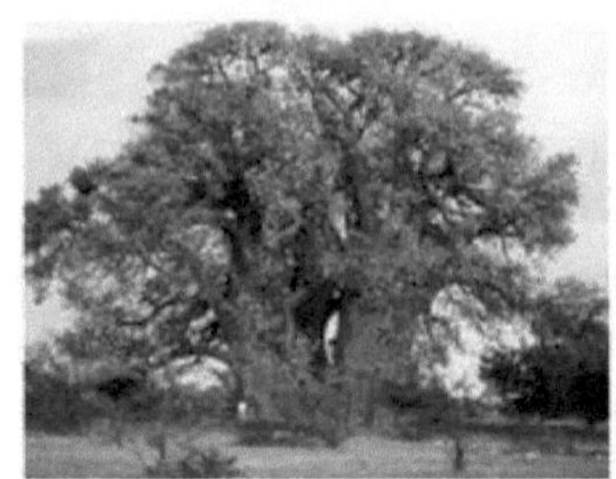

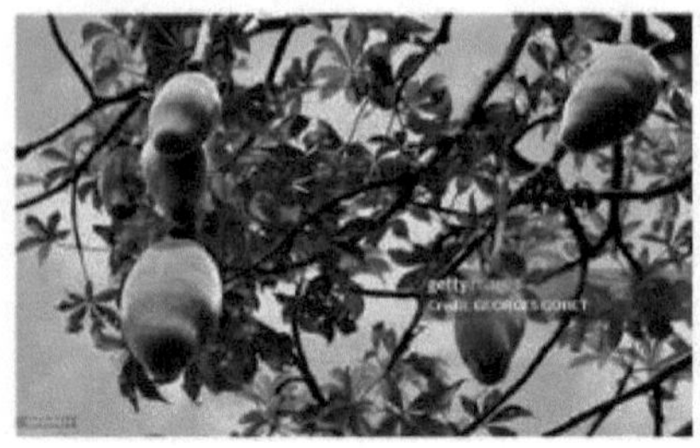

ACKNOWLEDGEMENTS

My sincere thanks to all you informants who spared no effort to open my mind to the unfathomable riches of natural medicine, the mysteries of which are usually said to be the preserve of the initiated. Thank you all for the great availability and honesty you have always shown, and the exquisite patience you have always shown at every meeting. My special thanks to you sirs:

AGOSSOU Nounagnon Marcel, lay exorcist in Cotonou AHLEGNAN Émile, traditional doctor in Calavi.

AHOUANGAN Koffi Lucien, traditional doctor, Banamè-Awolokpodji AKABASSI Benjamin, traditional doctor, Za-Kpota Centre

ALLINHLENON Sylvain, traditional doctor, specialist in fractures and dislocations in Tindji.

ATTINHOUHOU Thomas, traditional doctor in Za-Kpota Centre

AWONON Bienvenu, traditional doctor in Za-Kpota Centre

AWONON Pierre, traditional doctor in Za-Kpota Centre

Daa Bokonon Segan, traditional doctor, diviner, priest of Fa (Bokonon) in Affossogba

Daa Yanon: traditional healer and diviner priest of Fa (Bokonon) in Tindji GOGBE Elie, traditional doctor, specialist in mental illnesses in Davègo. HOUNNON GAHOU Miwakponhami, priest of the Vodun Thron and traditional doctor in Za-Kpota Centre.

HOUNON Pascal, traditional doctor in Za-Kpota centre

KPOHAZOUNDE Alain, Pastor of Celestial Christianity in Agondokpé

KOUDJÈ Thon Jérôme, traditional doctor in Za-Kpota Centre

KOUDJE Didier, traditional doctor at Za-Kpota Centre

KOUDJÈ Toussaint, traditional doctor, Za-Kpota Centre KPONHINTO Gérard, traditional doctor, Za-Kpota Centre LANGBEGNON Hervé, traditional doctor, Bohicon.

SONON Pascal, Evangelist of celestial Christianity in Za-Kékéré

DEDICATION

I dedicate this book to :

- *To all you professors, trainers and researchers in medicine, biochemistry, pharmacy, psychology, psychiatry, applied medical anthropology, ethnomedicine, pharmacopoeia and herbal medicine,*
- *To all you doctors and health workers who strive every day to save lives despite the sometimes difficult and difficult living and working conditions,*
- *To you men of God, bishops, priests, pastors and charismatics, to you religious institutions, who dedicate yourselves wholeheartedly to pastoral health care,*
- *To you, traditional doctors (Amawato) and diviners (Bokonon) and Vodoun priests (Vodounnon), who use our traditional holistic medical heritage in the service of life with responsibility and circumspection,*
- *To all you sick people around the world who are hoping for relief and healing,*
- *To men and women in search of the fullness of life.*
- *To all you young men and women who have helped and supported me in my investigations,*
- *To you, my dear parents Benjamin AKABASSI and Madeleine ZOUNKPEGANDJI, who very early on got me interested in the use of plants and their derivatives.*
- *To you, my sister Élisabeth AKABASSI, who are constantly with me in prayer as I embark on this bold research project for the well-being of every human being.*

INTRODUCTION

Adansonia digitata is known in French as *Baobab*, in Fon as *Kpassa*, in Nago as *Osché*, in Bariba as *Sônbu*, in Dendi as *Kôô*, in Ditamari as *Sônbu and Moutomu*, in Lokpa as *Télou,* in Bambara as *Sira*, in Peulh as *Babbe, Boki and Olohi*, and in Mandinke as *Sira and Sito*. In Sudanese Arabic in Kenya, it is called *Habhab*. In Tanzania, among the Masai, the baobab is called *Olimisera ol-unisera*; among the Chikwewa: *Mnambe, Mlambe*. In Mozambique, Somalia and Sudan, the tree is known in Arabic as *Tebeldi, Humr, Homeira*. It is one of the most highly recommended plants for medicinal treatments in tropical regions. The powder regulates digestive transit thanks to its fibre, which acts as a substrate for the intestinal microbiota and is effective against diarrhoea. It is a cholesterol-lowering agent, being accompanied by beta-sisterol, a phytocholesterol to reduce the absorption of dietary cholesterol. Thanks to its high vitamin C content, it helps regenerate vitamin E, contributes to energy metabolism, stimulates the body and improves the absorption of non-heme iron. Planter helps hemostatically to heal wounds. Its anti-poison properties are due to the alkaloid adansonine present in several parts of the tree. Baobab is an antipyretic and a protector of the osteo-articular system. It contributes to the formation of collagen, an essential protein that ensures the normal function of bones and cartilage, and is a component of blood vessel walls. It is an immunomodulator, a dental protector, a smoothing agent and a nervous system rebalancer, making collagen work, an essential protein for the oral cavity: the gums and teeth are richly made up of it. It helps to preserve the skin, contributes to the formation of neurotransmitters, stabilising the enzymes that synthesise the catecholamines that influence the functioning of the sympathetic nervous system, such as adrenalin and dopamine.

To rediscover the precious natural riches of the baobab, we're taking the following steps

to its study using a four-point descriptive method:

- Name and geographical distribution
- Botanical description
- Biochemical properties and therapeutic properties
- Toxicity

A botanical study of the plant and a botanical and phytomedical glossary will be added for greater understanding.

CHAPTER 1

1. Name and geographical distribution

Adansonia digitata (L.) is known in French as *Baobab, Arbre à palabres, Arbre-bouteille, Arbre du pharmacien, Arbre magique, Arbre de la vie.* In English: *Baobab, Dead-rat tree* , *Monkey-bread tree* , Upside-down *tree* , *Cream of tartar tree.* The name *Babobab*[1] derives from the Arabic *Bu- Hibab,* meaning *fruit with many seeds*. In Senegal, it is known in Wolof as *Goui* , *Gouis, Lalo, Bou* (tree), *Bui* (fruit), pulp (flour), *Gif* (seeds), *Tiega* (bark), *Lalo* (leaves), *Ndaba* (mucilage); in Sérer : *Bak, Mabk*; Niominka: *Bak, Ibak*; in Mading, Bambara, Malinké, Socé: *Sira, Sito*; in Malinké, Bambara: *Bavdi, Sirra, Boki*; in Chichewa: *Mnambe, mlambe*; in Nkonde: *Mbuye;* in Mandjaque: *Bedomhal, Bungal; in* Maure: *Téydum, Téyhum, Téyduma*; in Moré: *Trega, Twéga, Toayiga, Toéga*; Ndoute: *Ba*; in None, Safen: *Boh;* in Sarakolé: *Kidé*; in Foula, Peul, Poular, Tout-couleur: *Boy, Bohi, Boïo, Bokî, Boko, Bavdé, Babbe, Olohi, Boré*; in Senoufo: *Ngigne*; *Serer: Bâk, Mbak; Sonrai: Konian, Ko; in* Diola: *Bubak, Bubakabu, Buba* ; in Soussou: *Kiri*; Dogon: *Oro;* in Balanté: *Laté* ; in Mankagne: *Bedoal , Bedôgal, Bebak* ; in Bassai: *Anak* ; in Tandanké: *Anak, Ganak, Mamak, Gamak, Amak* . In Guinea, its name in Haousa is *Kuka*; in Djerma: *Ko.* In Côte d'Ivoire, it is known as *Fromdo* in Baoulé and *Ngigé* in Sénoufo. In Burkina Faso, it is called *Toyega* in Mossi, *Tuo* in Dagari and *Mor*[2] in Bisssa. In Benin, it is called in Fon: *Kpassatin*[3] ; in Nago: *Osché*; in Bariba: *Sônbu*; in Dendi: *Kôô*; in Ditamari: *Sônbu, Moutomu*; in Lokpa: *Télou.* The Malians call it in Dogon: *Oro*; in Bambara: *Sira*, in Peulh: *Babbe, Boki, Olohi*; in Mandinke: *Sira, Sito*; . In Sudanese Arabic in Kenya, it is called *Habhab.* In Tanzania, among the Masai, the baobab is called *Olimisera ol-unisera*; among the Chikwewa: *Mnambe, Mlambe*. In Mozambique, Somalia and Sudan, the tree is called *Tebeldi, Humr, Homeira* in Arabic (from Sudan); in Egypt and Ethiopia, it is called *Bamba* in Amhara; in Chad, it is called *Boki* by the Fulani and *Kuka* by the Haoussa. In Niger and Nigeria, it is called in Chad Arabic:

---

[1] There are two versions of the baobab in Africa. In one way, it is the title of the indigenous people of black Africa. Baobab means "bottle-shaped tree"; in another way, it is derived from an Arabic word. A long time ago, the pods of this tree were transported to Egypt, and the inhabitants didn't know what had happened. However, they found that the pod had many seeds, so the name "Bushebobu" means "fruit with many seeds". "Bushbob" later became "Baobobu". This dingy fruit looks like a loaf of bread, and monkeys and baboons love it. As a result, the tree's best-known name is Baobab. The tree's scientific name is little known, literally translated as "Adams finger".

[2] J Kerharo, "Le baobab, (Adansonia digitata), panacée africaine", *Quarterly Journal of Crude Drug Research:* 9/3 (1969) p. 1401-1408. Online publication 27/09 (2008).

[3] Our journalists Benjamin AKABASSI, Pierre AWONON and Daah Bokonon SEGAN, all traditional doctors.

Humar, Hamaraya, Hahar. In the Ivory Coast and Mali, it is known as Fromdo in Baoulé. In Zimbabwe, the baobab is known as Mwambo in Kamba, *Olimisera* in Masaï, *Muramba* in Mérou, *Umkhomo* in N'debele, *Mbuy in* N'Kondé, *Yag* in Somalia, *Mbuyu* in Swahili, *Hemmer, Dumma* in Tigre and *Mlonge* in Yao ([4]).
The name baobab was first mentioned in 1354 in the travel accounts of Ibn Battuta, the famous Arab explorer of the first half of the 14th century. Michel Adanson (1727-1806), after visiting Senegal in the mid-18th century, named the tree "baobab" after making a link with the fruit previously described by Alpino in 1592[5] . Subsequently, Carl Von Linné and Bernard de Jussieu named the tree *Adansonia digitata L.* in honour of Michel Adanson[6] .
In Africa, this species is found in semi-arid and sub-humid regions west of Madagascar and south of the Sahara, with the exception of Liberia, Uganda, Djibouti and Burundi. It is present in certain humid areas such as Benin, where rainfall exceeds 1,200 mm. In Chad, it is found only in the west and, in South Africa, it is essentially limited to the Transvaal[7] . In Senegal, it is found throughout the country, including the regions of Kaolack and Tambacounda, Fongolembi, Kédougou and Salémata, and the regions of Thiès, Louga, Matam and Saint-Louis. Exported outside Africa by Arab, French and Portuguese traders, it can be found in Asia (India, Indonesia, Sri Lanka, Malaysia, Java, the Philippines, Yemen, Iran and Taiwan), French Guiana, New Caledonia, Florida, Hawaii and the islands of Mauritius and Reunion[8] .

---

[4]Aïda Gabar DIOP et als, "Le baobab africain (Adansonia digitata L.) : principales caractéristiques et utilisations", *Fruits* 61/1 (2005) p.
55-69.
[5] G. E. Wickens, "The baobab: Africa's upside-down tree", *Kew Bulletin 37* (1982) p. 173-209.
[6] D. A. A Baum, "Systematic Revision of Adansonia (Bombacaceae)", *Annals of the Missouri Botanical Garden* 82 (1995) p. 440- 471.
[7] M. Sidibe et als, *Adansonia Digitata L. Fruits for the future 4. International Center for Underutilized Crops (ICUC): University of Southampton, Southampton*, UK 2002.
[8] A. Parsa, "Medicinal plants and drugs of plant origin in Iran", *Qualitas Plantarum et Materiae Vegetabiles* 5 (1959) p. 375- 394.

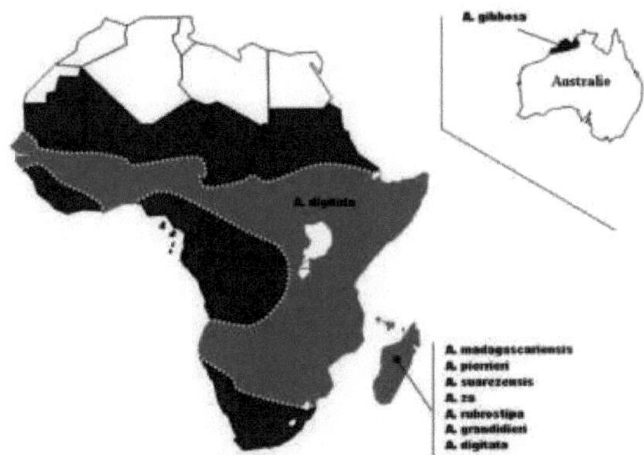

Distribution area of the eight baobab species in Africa, Madagascar and Australia. Adansonia fony and za seedlings are also grown. Countries where the genus Adansonia is present are shown in blue. The white boundary indicates the approximate area where baobab stands are most important in these same countries, with the northern limit corresponding to the Sahara.

The giant tree is found in the Sahelian, Sudano-Sahelian, Sudanian, Sudano-Guinean and Guinean zones, where the average annual rainfall is 300, 700, 800, 1100 and 1200 mm respectively[9] and where the average rainfall in these zones is less than 1,000 mm.

The average temperature varies from 24 (or sometimes lower) to 31°C and the air humidity from 18 to 99%[10] . It has been introduced into humid areas such as Gabon and the Democratic Republic of Congo (DRC)[11] . The baobab is better adapted to altitudes below 800 m, unlike its diploid ancestor *Adansonia kilima*, which was limited to altitudes of between 650 and 1,500 m in South Africa, Kenya, Namibia, Tanzania, Zambia and Zimbabwe[12] .

IUCN categories

[9] D. Sanogo et als, "Evaluation of fruit production of natural stands of Baobab (Adansonia digitata L.) in two climatic zones in Senegal", *Journal of Applied Biosciences* 85 (2015).

[10] A. E.Assogbadjo et als, "Caractères morphologiques et production des capsules de baobab (Adansonia digitata L.) au Bénin", *Fruits* 60 (2005) p. 327-340.

[11] A. E. Assogbadjo et als, *Adansonia digitata. African baobab. Conservation and sustainable use of genetic resources of priority food tree species in sub-Saharan Africa". Bioversity International*, Italy: 2011.

[12] C. Douie et als, "Verifying the presence of the newly discovered African baobab, Adansonia kilima, in Zimbabwe through morphological analysis", *South African Journal of Botany* 100 (2015) pp. 164-168.

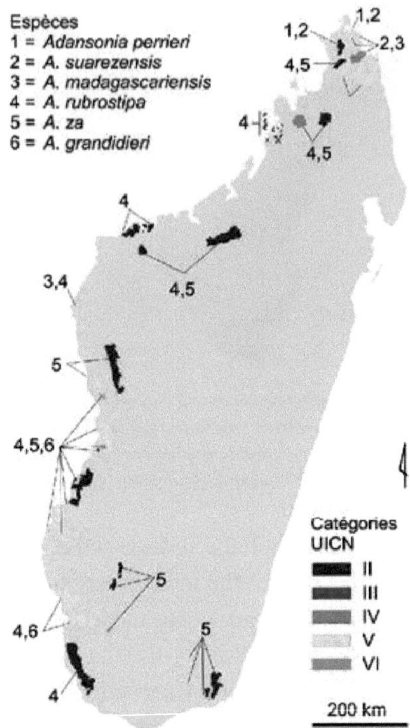

THE BAOBABS OF MADAGASCAR

Endemic baobab species in protected areas (IUCN categories: II = National Park, III = Natural Monument, IV = Special Reserve, V = Harmonious Protected Landscape, VI = Natural Resource Reserve)

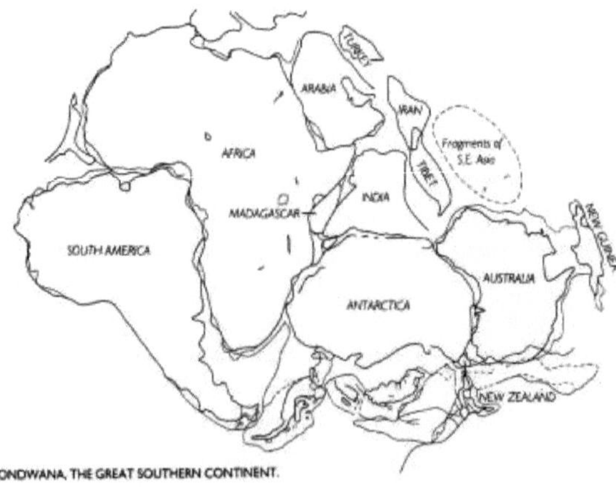

Boabs In The Kimberley | Geographical Distribution of the Boababs

Four morphotypes of baobab can be distinguished in Senegal according to the taste of the pulp, the size of the fruit, its resistance to breaking, the abundance of pulp and its colour. Malian farmers use the colour of the bark (black, red or grey), the taste of the pulp, the leaves, the colour of the seeds[13] and the shape of the capsules in Benin[14] as criteria. Other identification criteria are morphological variability and phenological variability[15] , using AFLP markers[16] (Amplified Fragments Length Polymorphism) of DNA (Deoxyribonucleic Acid) for baobabs in Benin, Burkina Faso, Ghana and Senegal[17] . In the west, the range extends from Cape Verde to the coastal plains of Ghana, Benin and Togo. In the north, it is bounded by the Sahara. In Eritrea and Somalia, the tree is typical of the plains, while in Sudan it grows in the Nuba mountains and at altitudes of up to 1,500 m in Ethiopia. In Kenya and further south towards Mozambique, populations are coastal or scattered in low-lying areas and savannah. In Angola and Namibia it tends to be found in wooded areas, while in Zimbabwe and northern South Africa[18] .

---

[13] M. Sidibe et als, *Baobab, Adansonia Digitata L. Fruits for the future 4. International Center for Underutilized Crops (ICUC)*: University of Southampton, Southampton, UK 2002.

[14] J. T. C Codjia et als, *Le baobab, une espèce à usage multiple au Bénin.* Cotonou, Benin, 2001.

[15] J. S. Jensen et als, "A research approach supporting domestication of Baobab (Adansonia digitata L.) in West Africa", *New Forests 41* (2011) p. 317-335.

[16] AFLP: Amplified fragment length polymorphism. AFLP is a non-locus-specific marker. It consists of PCR amplification of genomic DNA after digestion with two restriction enzymes and ligation of an adaptor of around 20 base pairs.

[17] T. Kyndt et als, "Spatial genetic structuring of baobab (Adansonia digitata, Malvaceae) in the traditional agroforestry systems of West Africa", *American Journal of Botany* 96 (2009) p. 950-957.

[18] Aïda Gabar Diop et als, "Le baobab africain (Adansonia digitata L.) : principales caractéristiques et utilisations", *Fruits* 61/1 (2005) p. 55-69.

CHAPTER 2

2. Botanical description

Adansonia digitata belongs to the *Bombacaceae* family and the *Malvales* order, in the same way as the kapok tree and the cheese tree[19] . The Adansonia genus consists of trees with mostly compact crowns, (5 to 30) m high, with trunks (2 to 10) m in diameter. The bark is grey or red. It is very fibrous on the inside. The soft wood is waterlogged and has a stratified structure.

The leaves are 2 to 7 cm wide, 5 to 16 cm long and 20 cm in diameter. They are alternate, digitate and deciduous in the dry season[20] and are petiolate (8 to 16 cm) and acuminate at the apex. A leaf may have between five and nine leaflets. The leaf blade, with a whole or denticulated margin, is usually glabrous and shiny on the upper side and slightly pubescent on the underside.

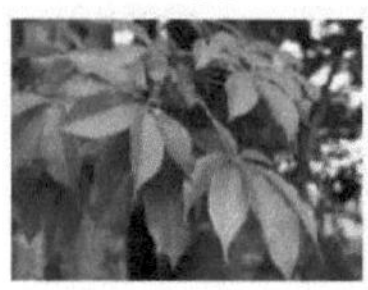
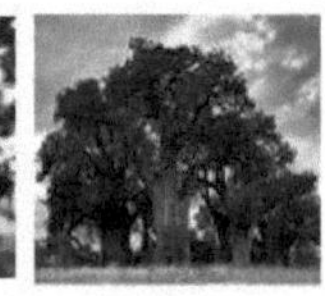
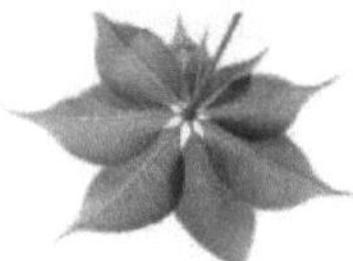
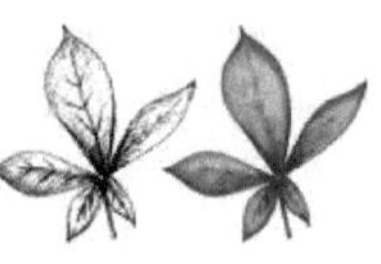

The flowers are white, sometimes greenish or brownish, 8 to 20 cm in diameter and hang from a stalk 15 cm to 1 m long. The baobab is the only species to have pendulous flowers, all the others being erect on a short stalk. The petals are oval, as wide as they are long, rounded at the tips and often slightly pubescent. They are deeply veined. The flowers have 700 to 1600 stamens and ovaries with five to ten cells. The flower bud is globose or oval and measures 5 to 7 cm in diameter. The apex is conical or apiculate.

Phenology is closely linked to the rainfall cycle. The flowering period varies enormously depending on location. In tropical climates, it generally takes place during the wet season: May to July in West Africa, October to December in the south of the continent and in Madagascar.

It is never seen at the height of the dry season. Flowering is gradual and takes place over several weeks.

---

[19] J. Kerharo et al, La pharmacopée sénégalaise traditionnelle - Plantes médicinales et toxiques, Vigot Frères, Paris, France, 1974.

[20] D. A. Zhigila et als, "A. Numericaò Taxinomy on Varieties of Adansonia Digitata L", *Annals. Food Science and Technology* 16 (2015) p. 157-167.

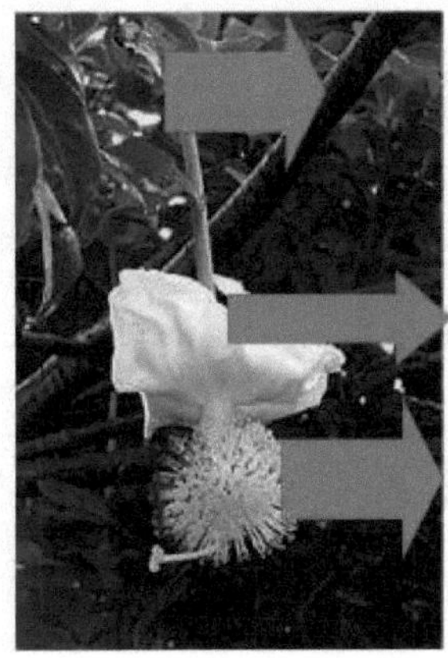

Peduncle
Petal
Infinite stamens
Baobab flower

The flowers, which are very short-lived, open at nightfall and remain open for only 16 to 20 hours, lasting only one night. The flower buds open in the early hours of the afternoon, open fully during the night and fade in the afternoon; the life cycle, therefore, does not exceed 24 hours. Pollination is mainly carried out by various fruit-eating megachiroptors (flying foxes) such as Eidolon helvum, Epomophorus gambianus and Rousettus aegyptiacus, which feed on the nectar and pollen of the flowers. The flowers emit a sour, sulphurous, even putrid scent that attracts these animals. Other vectors such as the wind, certain insects (ants, butterflies) or lemurs (in Madagascar) can also play a part. After pollination, the fruit takes 5 to 6 months to develop.

When they open, the calyx and corolla release some two thousand stamens, grouped together in a dense duster at the centre of which protrudes the curved style of the pistil.

They immediately emit a powerful scent that attracts bats, especially male fruit bats of the following species: the African spotted fruit bat (Eidolon helvum), the Egyptian spotted fruit bat (Rousettes aepyptiacus) and Wahlberg's spotted fruit bat (Epomorphorus wahlbergi), which enjoy the abundant nectar for two months.

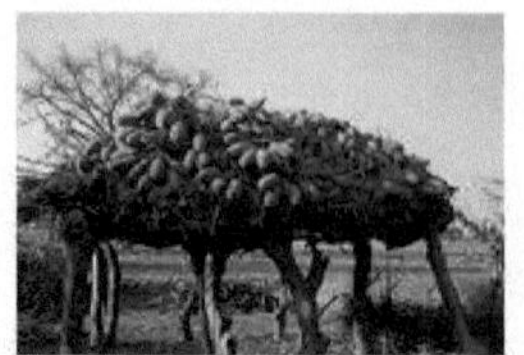
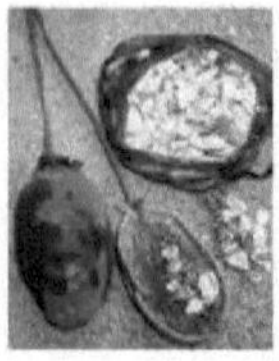
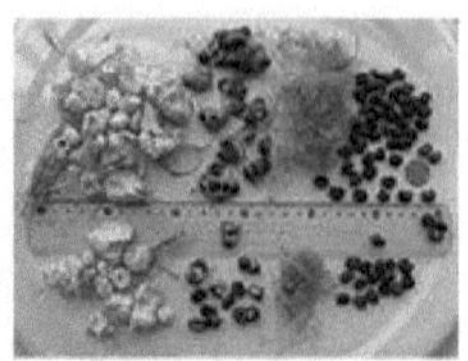

Fruit drying in Senegal Open fruit with seeds Pulp and seeds

The indehiscent fruit falls from the tree when ripe without opening immediately. The pulp is usually eaten by termites, which penetrate the fruit and release hard, black, bean-shaped seeds. If they do not germinate *in situ*, the seeds are dispersed by monkeys, rats, elephants, birds and humans, who are also major consumers of the fruit.

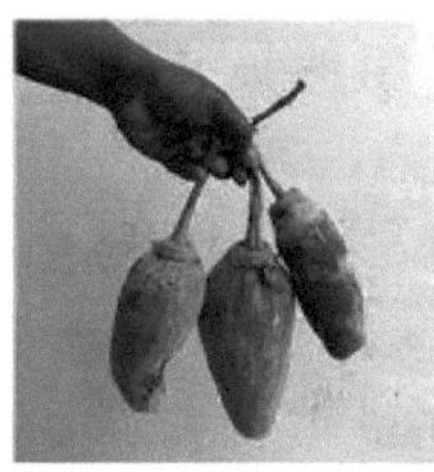

The fruit is a capsule attached to a long stem with a hard, woody pod 20 to 30 cm long. It is generally ovoid, spherical, fusiform, elongated or club-shaped, measuring 7 to 20 cm by 7 to 54 cm. In Benin, the length can vary from 16.32 to 21.42 cm and the width from 8.3 to 9.6 cm[21] . The capsule pericarps are much thinner (0.4 to 0.5 cm) than those usually found in other parts of Africa, which are 0.8 to 1 cm. The fruit is sometimes apiculate, pointed or rounded at the tip, with a brownish, yellowish or greenish downy surface. It can weigh over 496 g in Niger. It contains 2,000 to 3,000 seeds per kg, surrounded by a floury white or yellow pulp and mixed with reddish fibres[22] . In Senegal, the average fruit production per individual of Adansonia digitata is 35.5 kg of fruit in the Sudano-Sahelian zone and 64.9 kg of fruit in the SudanoGuinean zone, with 468.6 kg.ha and 558.14 kg.ha respectively[23] . In Benin, a boll weighs 275 g in the Guinean zone, 273 g in the Sudano-Guinean zone and 204 g in the Sudanian zone. In each of these zones, it produces 54g, 51g and 32g of pulp respectively, as well as 37g, 28g and 23g of kernels. The weight of the kernels and the thickness of the capsule endocarp in the Guinean zone are greater than those in the Sudanian

[21] A. E. Assogbadjo et als, "Caractères morphologiques et production des capsules de baobab (Adansonia digitata L.) au Bénin", *Fruits* 60 (2005) p. 327-340.

[22] A. E. Assogbadjo et als, p. 327-340.

[23] D. Sanogo et als, "Evaluation of fruit production of natural stands of Baobab (Adansonia digitata L.) in two climatic zones in Senegal", *Journal of Applied Biosciences* 85 (2015).

and Sudano-Guinean zones[24] . In Sudan and Kenya, the average number of fruits per baobab in Kordofan in Sudan is 381, while in Kibwezi in Kenya, the averages vary from 360 to 707 fruits[25] . Trees that produce a lot of fruit are now classified as "female", while those that produce almost no fruit are called male[26] . In its natural state, the thick seed coat takes three to five years to decompose and allow the seed to germinate, but this can be reduced to a few days by scarifying the seed coat and then immersing the seed in water.

The bark is smooth, grey/silver to brown and purple in colour and can be up to 10 cm thick.

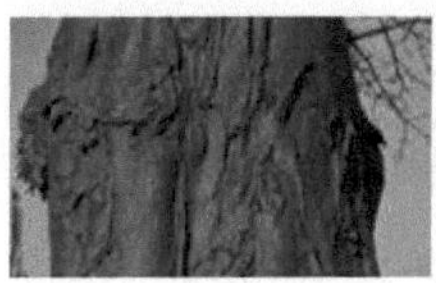
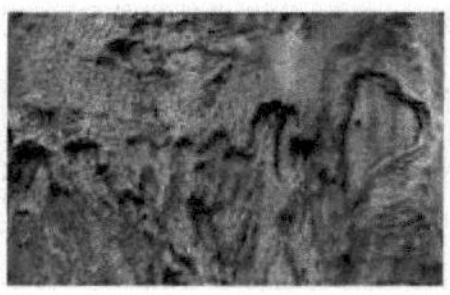
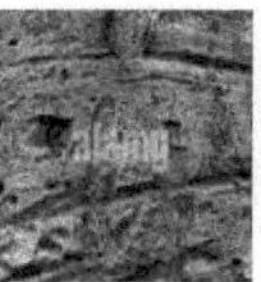
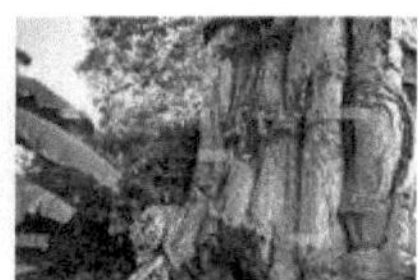

Baobab bark

[24]A. E. Assogbadjo et als, p. 327-340.

[25]B. K .Sharma et als, "Adansonia digitata L. (Malvaceae) a threatened tree species of medicinal impor tance", *Medicinal Plants - International Journal of Phytomedicines and Related Industries* / (2015) p. 173.

[26] S. M. Venter et als, "Baobab (Adansonia digitata L.) fruit production in communal and conservation landuse types in Southern Africa", *Forest Ecology and Management* 261 (2011) p. 630-639.

The bark fibres are usually torn from the lowest parts of the trunk and despite this rather cruel technique, which is fatal to other plants, the baobab survives and produces new bark. The most resistant fibres are used in various fields (ropes, reins, strings for musical instruments, baskets, nets, fishing line, fibres for fabrics).

The trunk can be conical, cylindrical, bottle-shaped or short and thick, reaching up to 10/12 metres in diameter. With its spongy tissues, it is always able to accumulate liquids, allowing the plant to store water during the rainy season and conserve it for the dry season, thus becoming a water reserve for both people and animals living in the surrounding area. When large, the tree can hold up to 9,000 litres of water and sometimes more than 100,000 litres in its trunk, enabling many sedentary communities and nomadic tribes such as the Kalahari bushmen to

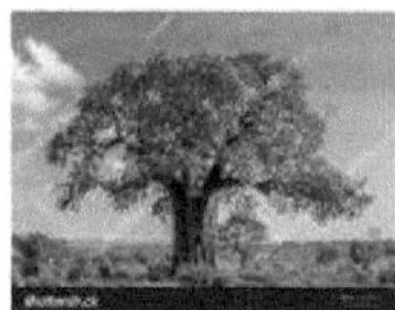

survive, even when far from any water source. These populations use hollow stems joined together like straws to reach the water inside the trunk. The populations of certain dry regions in Sudan, such as Kordofan and Darfur, have transformed certain baobabs into veritable wells or cisterns, without them dying out. The baobab is dug out from the top down to ground level, with a vast funnel with a very gentle slope all around the tree so that water concentrates around the trunk when it rains. The top is then blocked with branches and clay when the cistern is filled during the rainy season.

A tap is installed at the base, so that in times of drought you can enjoy fresh, pure water with a pleasant lemony taste[31] .

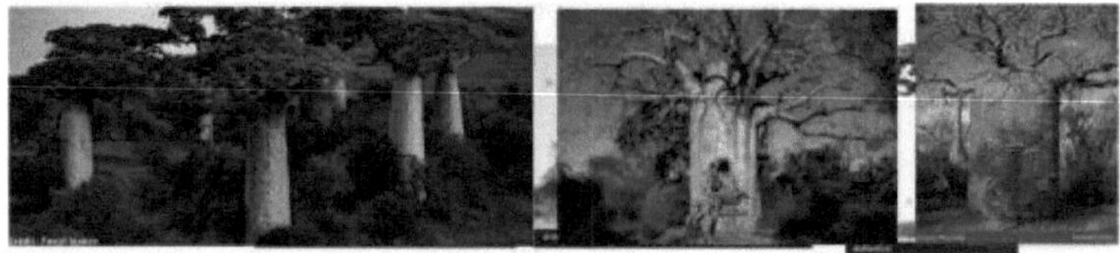

Water storage trunks

In West Africa, the hollow trunk can be used as a prison, stable or storehouse, and in Zimbabwe as a waiting room for buses.

31 "Le baobab en Afrique, plus qu'un symbole, une ressourc. e : l'arbre aux mille usages", *Futura* , accessed 17/04/2024 (https://www.futura-sciences.com/planete/dossiers/botanique-baobab-arbre-pharmacien-arbre- vie-666/page/6/) p. 1-8.

30/40 individuals. The branches form a wide crown and taper towards the ends; the young branches are voluminous and rarely hairless.

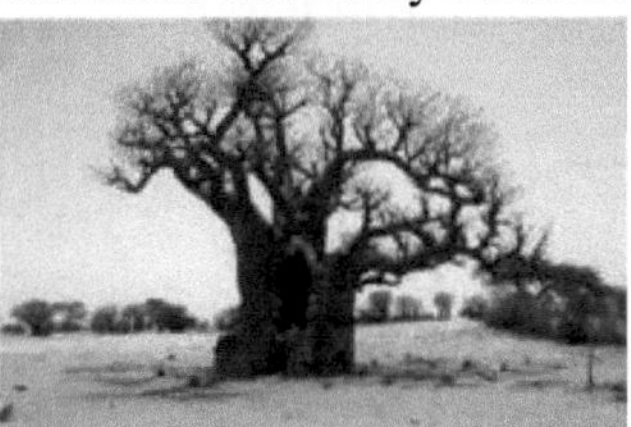

The cavernous trunk as a waiting room with slender branches at the ends forming a crown

The baobab has a fairly extensive lateral root system. The rootlets can extend up to 50 m from the trunk and 10 m deep. The main roots rarely extend more than a few metres and remain superficial. Some of them are tuberised at the tip.

Nine of the thirteen oldest baobabs in Africa, aged between 1,100 and 2,500 years, have died in the last decade, probably as a result of climate change. The oldest baobab in France is located on the island of Mayotte, and is over 400 years old.[28]

[28]) Adrian Patrut et als, "Age and architecture of the largest African Baobabs from Mayotte, France", DRC Sustainable Future*: Journal of Environment, Agriculture, and Energy* 1 (2020) p. 33-47 (DOI 10.37281/DRCSF/1.1.5).

CHAPTER 3

3. Biochemical properties and phytotherapeutic properties

Baobab's natural composition contains 18 amino acids, 8 of which are essential: proline, histidine, threonine, tryptophan, phenylalanine, valine, methionine, leucine, lysine, tyrosine; vitamins: A, B1, B2, B3, C; minerals and trace elements: calcium, copper, iron, potassium, magnesium, manganese, sodium, phosphorus, zinc; fatty acids : oleic acid, linoleic acid, palmitic acid, stearic acid; carotenoid: lutein; natural acids: citric acid, tartaric acid, malic acid, succinic acid; antioxidants: procyanidins, flavonoids; proteins; carbohydrates; fibre; sugars: fructose, sucrose, glucose; pectins. The fruit consists of 14-28% pulp, which is low in water, acidic, starchy and rich in vitamin C, calcium and magnesium.

Leaves are considered to be a source of micronutrients required for metabolic functions[29] . Dried, they are rich in protein (8.00 ± 0.90%), lipids (15.93 ± 0.62%) and carbohydrates (61.60 ± 0.69%)[30] , mucilage (12%)[31] vitamin C, i.e. 14.98 mg.100g[32] from leaves dried at room temperature and collected in Nigeria. They are also rich in essential amino acids[33] and minerals, the most common of which are sodium (Na), magnesium (Mg), calcium (Ca), potassium (K) and iron (Fe)[34] . They are also rich in flavonoids (catechin, epicatechin, rutin, quercetin, campferol, luteolin) and phenolic acids (caffeic acid, chlorogenic acid, gallic acid and ellagic acid). The methanolic extract of the leaves has antioxidant activity and an inhibitory effect on the enzymatic activities (α-amylase, α-glucosidase and aldose reductase) linked to type 2 diabetes (T2DM). In addition

---

[29] C. C. Ogbaga et als, *Phytochemical, Elemental and Proximate Analyses of Stored, Sun-Dried and Shade- Dried Baobab (Adansonia Digitata)* Leaves. 2017

[30] O. P. Edogbanya, "Comparative Study of the Proximate Composition of Edible Parts of Adansonia digitata L. obtained from Zaria, Kaduna State, Nigeria. MAYFEB", *Journal of Biology and Medicine* 1 (2016).

[31] R. Gaiwe et als, "Calcium and mucilage in the leaves of Adansonia digitata (Baobab)", *International Journal of Crude Drug Research 27 (*1989,) p. 101-104.

[32] D. Abiona et als, "Proximate Analysis, Phytochemical Screening and Antimicrobial Activity of Baobab (Adansonia digitata) Leaves", . *IOSR JAC 8 (*2015) p. 60-65.

[33] T. Hyacinthe et als, "Variability of vitamins B1, B2 and minerals content in baobab (Adansonia digitata) leaves in East and West Africa ", *Food Science & Nutrition* 3 (2015) p. 3, 17-24.

[34] V. F. Abioye et als, "Effects of different drying methods on the nutritional and quality attributes of baobab leaves (Adansonia digitata)", *Agric. Biol. J. N. Am 5 (*2014) p. 104-108.

Allossekpínmánssín or the prospect of health gained for all phenolic compound content of fresh and blanched leaves respectively at 20.02 ± 1.83 mgGAE.g and 16.80 ± 1.02 mgGAE.g. Analyses in 2017[35] revealed 17 compounds, the majority of which are squalene (27.06%) and phytol (13.28%). The minotaries are: palmitic acid (8.95%), α-amyrin (7.02%), octacosane (5.26%), nonacosane (5.05%), γ-sitosterol (4.98%), germanicol (4.08%) and friedelin (3.60%).

The pulp contains most of the elements found in the seeds, which generally have a higher content. It represents between 13 and 25% of the total mass of the fruit[36] . Its water content is low, between 6 and 28%[37] due to low annual rainfall, high moderate temperatures, low altitude and exposure to sun and wind. It is also rich in pectin[38] , sugar (between 7.2 and 11.8 g of glucose equivalent per 100 g of dry pulp)[39] , fructose, glucose and sucrose[40] . The total sugar content is 23.2% and the reducing sugar content is 18.9%[41] . The high titratable acidity content ranges from 68 to 201 mEq.100 g. This acidity is due to the presence of organic acids such as citric acid, tartaric acid, malic acid, succinic acid, pyruvic acid, fumaric acid and 3- hydroxybutanoic acid[42] .

But citric acid is most abundant in the pulp. The pulp is also rich in protein, the level of which depends on the soil and climate conditions[43] . It is also rich in minerals ranging from 3.7 to 6.3%[44] : potatium, calcium between 250 and 655

---

[35]M. B. Suliman, et als, "Chemical Composition and Antibacterial Activity of Crude Extracts from Sudanese Medicinal Plant Adansonia digitata L", *Chemistry of Advanced Materials 2* (2017) p. 2

[36] M. Cisse et als, "Caractérisation du fruit du baobab et étude de sa transformation en nectar", *Fruits 64 (*2009) p. 64, 19-34.

[37] P. Soloviev et als, "Variabilité des caractères physico-chimiques des fruits de trois espèces ligneuses de cueillette récoltés au Sénégal: Adansonia digitata , Balanites aegyptiaca et Tamarindus indica", *Fruits* 59 (2004,) p. 109-119.

[38] A. A. Nour et als, "Chemical composition of baobab fruit (Adansonia digitata L.)", *Tropical Science* 22 (1980) p. 383-388.

[39] P. Soloviev et als, "Variabilité des caractères physico-chimiques des fruits de trois espèces ligneuses de cueillette récoltés au Sénégal: Adansonia digitata. Balanites aegyptiaca et Tamarindus indica", *Fruits* 59 (2004) p. 109-119.

[40] M. Cisse "Characterisation of baobab fruit and study of its transformation into nectar", *Fruits* 64 (2009) p. 19-34.

[41] A. A. Nour et als, "Chemical composition of baobab fruit (Adansonia digitata L.)", . *Tropical Science* 22 (1980) p. 383-388.

[42] B. Khakimov et als, "A comprehensive and comparative GC-MS metabolomics study of non-volatiles in Tanzanian grown mango, pineapple, jackfruit, baobab and tamarind fruits",. *Food Chemistry* 213 (2016) p.
691-699.

[43] M. A.Osman, "Chemical and nutrient analysis of baobab (Adansonia digitata) fruit and seed protein solubility", *Plant Foods for Human Nutrition (Formerly Qualitas Plantarum)* 59 (2004) p. 29-33 .

[44] A. A. Nour et als, "Chemical composition of baobab fruit (Adansonia digitata L.)",

mg.100g[45] , magnesium and phosphorus between 96 and 210 mg.100g[46] , iron between 14 and 76 mg.kg, copper, zinc and manganese. The pulp is a good source of essential elements (Cu, Ca, Fe, K, Mn, Zn) in addition to 10 new elements identified[47] . Trace levels of heavy metals (As, Cd, Hg) are below limit values. The pulp also contains the vitamins ascorbic acid (vitamin C), with a content of between 200 and 500 mg.100 g, a content often due to the soil and climate conditions of the tree, the stage of ripeness of the fruit at harvest and the storage conditions of the pulp[48] . The β-carotene content is between 2.16 ± 1.77 and 3.16 ± 1.68 mg.100g[49] . The antioxidant power of the pulp is estimated at 88 µmol trolox.g[50] . This content is probably due to the high ascorbic acid content. Total polyphenols are estimated at 63.56 ± 0.79 mg/g EAG[51] . The pulp is also rich in vitamins B1, B2, B6 and A in significant quantities[52] . There are also amino acids such as alanine, arginine (7.6%), glycine, lysine, methionine, proline, serine and valine[53] , tyrosine (20.6%) and glutamic acid (6.5%). Very recently, four (4) hydroxycinnamic acid glycosides, six (6) iridoid glycosides and three (3) phenylethanoid glycosides have been identified. Hydroxycinnamic acids, natural antioxidants present in fruit, vegetables and cereals, have anti-carcinogenic, anti-microbial and anti-inflammatory properties[54] . It is important to note that the variation in fruit composition is caused by the environment, the type of soil, the water or the intensity of the sun[55] .

---

*Tropical Science 22 (*1980) p. 383-388.

[45]A. A. Nour et als, p. 383-388.

[46] M. Sidibe et als, *Baobab, Adansonia Digitata L. Fruits for the future 4. International Center for Underutilized Crops (ICUC):* University of Southampton, Southampton, UK 2002.

[47] I. K. Baidoo et als, "Major, Minor and Trace Element Analysis of Baobab Fruit and Seed by Instrumental Neutron Activation Analysis Technique", *Food and Nutrition Sciences* 04 (2013) pp. 772-778.

[48] M. A. Osman, "Chemical and nutrient analysis of baobab (Adansonia digitata) fruit and seed protein solubility", *Plant Foods for Human Nutrition (Formerly Qualitas Plantarum) 59 (*2004) p. 29-33.

[49] A. E. Aluko, et als, "Nutritional Quality and Functional Properties of Baobab (Adansonia digitata) Pulp from Tanzania", *Journal of Food Research* 5/23 (2016).

[50] M. Cisse et als, "Caractérisation du fruit du baobab et étude de sa transformation en nectar", *Fruits* 64 (2009) p. 19-34.

[51] E. O. Kim et als, "Anti-inflammatory activity of hydroxycinnamic acid derivatives isolated from corn bran in lipopolysaccharide-stimulated Raw 264.7 macrophages", *Food and Chemical Toxicology* 50 (2012) pp. 1309-1316.

[52] G. P. P. Kamatou et als, "An updated review of Adansonia digitata: A commercially important African tree", *South African Journal of Botany 77* (2011) pp. 908-919.

[53]G. P. P. Kamatou, pp. 908-919.

[54] C.-J. Weng et al, "Chemopreventive effects of dietary phytochemicals against cancer invasion and metastasis: Phenolic acids, monophenol, polyphenol, and their derivatives", *Cancer Treatment Reviews* 38 (2012) p. 76-87.

[55]A. E. Assogbadjo et als, "Variation in biochemical composition of baobab (Adansonia

Baobab pulp is particularly rich in antioxidants: vitamin A, vitamin C, procyanidins, flavonoids and carotenoids, all compounds that fight free radicals and prevent cell damage. The procyanidins contained in baobab fruit pulp are tannins found in certain fruits, such as grapes and apples, and in cocoa. They are renowned for their ability to eliminate free radicals and for their effectiveness in preventing oxidative stress.

The parts most commonly used in food are the fruit pulp, the leaves and the seeds. The pulp is used to make nectar-type drinks (fruit pulp with added water and sugar), sauces, food supplements and Ngalax during religious festivals such as Korité and Easter. Ngalax is a sweet liquid mixture made from peanut paste, baobab fruit pulp and cooked rolled millet flour. The young leaves can be eaten raw or boiled. The powder of dried and sieved baobab leaves, called Lalo in Senegal, is used as a binder in millet couscous or to flavour sauces. The seeds can be eaten fresh or dried[56] , roasted and consumed as a coffee substitute[57] . The ground seeds are used as a thickener for sauces and soups. The condiment obtained after fermentation and air-drying of the seeds is used in traditional cooking as a source of protein or flavour enhancer in soups and stews[58] . It is called Maari in Burkina Faso, Dikouanyouri (or Tayohunta from almonds) in Benin, N'Gono in Mali and Dadawa (or Issai) in Nigeria[59] . The almond sauce obtained by grinding the roasted seeds is also used as a tomato paste or spicy sauce[60] .

Traditional therapies use the leaves, bark, roots, seeds, fruit pulp and flowers. Today, clinical studies have revealed their antisickling, antibacterial, antidiabetic, antirheumatic, antitrypanosome, arthritic, anti-inflammatory, antimicrobial, antioxidant, antiviral, analgesic, antipyretic, diuretic and

---

digitata) pulp, leaves and seeds in relation to soil types and tree provenances", *Agriculture, Ecosystems & Environment* 157 (2012) pp. 157, 94-99.

[56] G. A Wickens, *The Uses of the Baobab (Adansonia digitata L.) in Africa. In: Browse in Africa.* ILRI (aka ILCA and ILRAD): Addis-Ababa, Ethiopia 1980.

[57] N.Salih et al., "Phenolics and fatty acids compositions of vitex and baobab seeds used as coffee substitutes in Nuba Mountains, Sudan", *Agriculture And Biology Journal Of North America* 6 (2015) p. 90-93.

[58] C. Parkouda, et als, "The microbiology of alkaline-fermentation of indigenous seeds used as food condiments in Africa and Asia", *Critical Reviews in Microbiology 35 (*2009) p. 139-156.

[59] C. Parkouda et al, "Biochemical changes associated with the fermentation of baobab seeds in Maari: An alkaline fermented seeds condiment from western Africa", *Journal of Ethnic Foods* 2 (2015) p. 58-63. Cf F. J. Chadare et als, "Indigenous Knowledge and Processing of Adansonia Digitata L. Food Products in Benin", *Ecology of Food and Nutrition* 47 (2008) p. 338-362.

[60] F. J. Chadare et als, "Baobab Food Products: A Review on their Composition and Nutritional Value", *Critical Reviews in Food Science and Nutrition* 49 (2009) p. 254-274.

hepatoprotective activities[61] .

Despite a lysine deficiency and the presence of a number of anti-constitutional factors, seeds are an interesting source of protein. They contain around 15% lipids. After cooking or roasting, they are eaten directly or used as a thickener in powder form. The leaves are rich in vitamins (particularly C and A) and iron, and contain mucilage (10% ms). The youngest leaves can be eaten as a vegetable, but more commonly they are dried and then ground into a powder[66] .

The pulp of the fruit is an onifiant/stimulant, antidiarrhoeal, antienteralgic, antipyretic, haemostatic/healing and aphrodisiac. Its extracts are effective against fatigue, inappetence, diarrhoea, enteralgia (especially in children), malaria, nasopharyngeal infections, circulatory disorders (haemorrhoids), haemoptysis and insect bites. To treat dermatitis, powder old, charred fruit hulls and mix 3 pinches of the powder with cow's butter. The mixture should be applied regularly to all parts of the skin affected by the rash, healing within a few days. To treat incurable wounds, the hull should be calcined and pulverised. The wounds are then washed and covered with one or two pinches of the powder. Each dressing should last 2 or 3 days before being cleaned. If the wound is not very deep, it will heal within a few days. In the case of panicitis, the treatment consists of mixing 3 pinches of the calcined old hull powder with cow's butter to obtain a pasty mixture. The mixture obtained in the treatment of dermatitis is used to cover the affected finger, at a rate of 7 to 10 applications, i.e. one application per day. After 7 applications, the pain is completely relieved. And when it comes to treating ringworm and the external deworming of animals, the calcined shell must be crushed to obtain a powder which is mixed with ointment to obtain a pasty mixture. This mixture is applied regularly until the pimples or parasites have disappeared. However, the hair must first be shaved and the pasty mixture applied to the animal's entire body. Its anti-inflammatory and antioxidant properties protect and repair the liver.

The pulp of the baobab fruit has a high vitamin C (or ascorbic acid) content, with 373 mg per 100g. It therefore contains 7 times more vitamin C than lemons (50 mg per 100g) and 6 times more than oranges (57 mg per 100g). Ascorbic acid is the energy and vitality vitamin par excellence. It boosts the immune system, improves iron absorption and fights free radicals. Other components of the pulp also have an invigorating effect. These include carbohydrates and

[61] S. Singh et als, "Medicinal uses of adansonia digitata l.: an endangered tree species", *Journal of Pharmaceutical and Scientific Innovation* 2 (2013) pp. 14-16. Cf M. Yusha'u et als, "Antibacterial activity of Adansonia digitata stem bark extracts on some clinical bacterial isolates", *International Journal of Biomedical and Health Sciences 6* (2010) p. 129-135. Cf A. A. Al-Qarawi et als, "Hepatoprotective Influence of Adansonia digitata Pulp", *Journal of Herbs, Spices & Medicinal Plants* 10 (2003) p. 1-6.

lipids, which are our body's main sources of energy, and vitamin B2 (riboflavin), which is involved in energy metabolism. Thanks to these different components, baobab fruit pulp is ideal for people who are tired or convalescing, or for preventing winter ailments (colds, flu, etc.) by boosting the immune system. The University of Abomey-Calavi in Benin conducted a laboratory study which revealed the high vitamin C content of the pulp[62] .

The seed is antidiarrhoeal and enteralgic. It combats hypertension, coughs and malaria. It stimulates lactation, relieves hiccups and fights gingivitis and mouth infections. In Benin, seed kernels are used to soothe hiccups. They are crushed and served with a teaspoon of the product diluted in a glass of water or milk. The potion is particularly recommended for children. stomach aches. The pulp is recommended for ulcers and loss of virility. It is a tonic and stimulant, for convalescence, malaria, inappetence, diarrhoea, colds and coughs, flu and haemorrhoids. However, excess pulp can lead to constipation.

The leaves are effective against haemorrhoids, enteralgia and teething pains in infants. It activates perspiration and combats rheumatism, conjunctivitis, otitis, urinary tract infections, insect bites, dracunculiasis and skin inflammation. The leaf powder is used to treat internal haemorrhoids. The mixture must be properly beaten to obtain a homogeneous, concentrated, sticky mixture, which the patient should drink at a rate of 3 tablespoons in a quarter litre of water, to be taken in a single dose and repeated for 3 days during the week. The treatment may last several weeks or even months, depending on the extent of the illness. To combat constipation in cattle, you need ½ kg of leaf powder in 2 litres of water, stirring vigorously until you obtain a homogeneous, concentrated mixture. The dosage is 1 litre of the mixture administered through a hose for 2 days. In the case of constipation in humans, it is advisable to beat the solution thoroughly until a homogeneous, concentrated, sticky mixture is obtained, which the patient is given to drink at a rate of 3 tablespoons in a quarter litre of water, to be consumed in a single dose. The patient is deconstipated within two or three hours. It is possible to have pasty stools and buzzing in the stomach for a few hours.

As for the bark, it is an antipyretic. It is effective against fever, malaria, diarrhoea and inflammation of the digestive tract. It is a tonic for young children. It relieves lumbago, menorrhagia, toothache, ulcers and other complaints.

---

[62] Juia Perez, "Baobab, the pharmacist's tree", Darwin Nutrition 8/12 (2022) p. 1-6.
Aidda Gabar Diop, *The African baobab (Adansonia digitata L.): main characteristics and uses* Cambridge University Press, (2006).

burns. It is used to treat superficial wounds and to soften the skin. The fresh bark is crushed in a small quantity of water until a substrate is obtained to heal circumcision wounds, sprinkled on a daily basis for a week. The wound must be left in contact with the air.

The root is a tonic, stimulant and fortifier. It is effective against malaria, epilepsy and agalactia (often in combination with other plants). The flowers act as a tonic and combat malaria, epilepsy and agalactia (often in combination with other plants). It facilitates childbirth and combats coughs and anaemia.

Baobab oil can be combined with shea and coconut oils to treat dry, brittle hair. It also makes hair supple and shiny. Applying the paste obtained by crushing the seeds as a hair mask effectively prevents dandruff and other scalp infections. It also has a moisturising and softening effect on the skin. In fact, like shea oil, it is used to care for the skin, especially children's skin. It is highly recommended during periods of extreme cold and the dry seasons to prevent damage to skin cells. It is also a valuable antioxidant. The seeds and pulp can be incorporated into soap, exfoliating masks and ointments. Thanks to their emollient properties, they keep the skin smooth and silky. Baobab is also used in many anti-ageing products, as well as in hair care.

The leaves and seeds can be used to heal an external wound by applying the gum to disinfect it; the leaves must then be rubbed together and the juice extracted to heal the wound, twice a day. The paste obtained by crushing the seeds is mainly used for burns. The fibres extracted from the pulp are used as a sponge to wash patients and soothe itching. Baobab is used to treat osteoarthritis and polyarthritis. Baobab pulp contains twice as much calcium as a glass of milk. Phosphorus and calcium are essential for healthy bones. Their intake is essential for the body, particularly for people suffering from osteoarthritis or polyarthritis. Very rich in potassium, baobab helps the entire muscular system to function properly. Its analgesic effect also helps to better manage the consequences of these two diseases. To cure fever and malaria, drink an infusion or decoction of baobab. It is recommended for its anti-inflammatory and anti-oxidant properties for people suffering from cancer, auto-immune diseases and various other inflammatory diseases. It also protects the liver. And thanks to its essential contribution of good bacteria, it combats intestinal inflammation. It is a natural fortifier, thanks to its high content of organic acids, calcium and vitamins. The leaves contain a high concentration of proteins and calcium, while the seeds are rich in trace elements and various other vitamins, making it an inexhaustible source of energy. All parts of the tree can be consumed as powders, drinks, herbal teas or decoctions. Baobab is highly effective against stomach ailments thanks to its content of organic acids, mainly citric and tartaric acids. These include dysentery, diarrhoea and inflammation of the digestive tract, as well as dehydration caused by these gastric ailments. Its fibre content also helps to maintain the digestive system[63] .

Both the leaves and the pulp are valuable allies in inflammatory conditions such as osteoarthritis and rheumatoid arthritis. In fact, as well as relieving joint pain, baobab reduces inflammation, in the same way as turmeric. This action is largely due to the presence of methionine, proline, polyphenols and vitamins that help reduce cytokines, substances that encourage inflammation. In particular, vitamin A or retinol acts on the inflammatory mediator MCP-1 (monocyte chemoattractant protein 1), which is involved in a number of diseases such as rheumatoid arthritis. Group B vitamins also play an important role in reducing inflammation in the joints. As for methionine and proline, these are amino acids that contribute to the formation of cartilage.

The macerated and compressed leaves can be used to clean the ears and eyes of sick children, with an anti-inflammatory effect. In traditional medicine, the leaves are used for their expectorant, febrifuge, hypotensive and anti-asthmatic properties, and to control excessive perspiration. The leaves are also used to treat urinary tract diseases, diarrhoea, inflammations and insect bites. They are also an effective remedy for expelling guinea worms. They can also be used outdoors, thanks to their anti-oxidant and emollient properties, which make the skin supple and elastic.

Baobab is also renowned for its analgesic action. This property is found not only in the pulp but also in the bark of the tree, consumed as an infusion or decoction. It relieves muscle and joint pain, and also helps to reduce inflammation. In this sense, its properties are similar to those of another tree, boswellia. Group B vitamins, vitamin C, phenylalanine and histidine are responsible for this pain-relieving action. Phenylalanine, for example, is an essential amino acid involved in reducing pain, including chronic pain. It does this by inhibiting the activity of enkephalinase, a brain enzyme that amplifies pain signals. The study conducted on rats by the University of Ilorin (Nigeria) demonstrates the analgesic effect of African baobab bark extract[64] .

Thanks to its lubricating and diluting properties and the presence of pectins and carbohydrates, Baobab pulp has recently been used as a hydrophilic base for pharmaceutical formulations of long-acting paracetamol and theophylline tablets.

In Sierra Leone, the root stimulates sexual activity. Dried root powder prepared as a cream is used as a tonic for malaria sufferers. In Zambia, an infusion of the

---

[63] INECOBA, "12 medicinal properties of baobab", *INECOBA* 17/06 (2015) p. 1-2.

[64] Juia Perez, "Baobab, the pharmacist's tree", Darwin Nutrition 8/12 (2022) p. 1-6.

roots is used in children's baths to make the skin smooth and supple.
The pulp can be chewed and swallowed, or dissolved in water or condensed milk to make a refreshing, high-energy drink known in Senegal as "bouye". This drink is sometimes mixed with "mérissa", a type of fermented sorghum beer very common in Sudan. Finally, in some parts of Africa, baobab pulp is burnt to fumigate insects that parasitise domestic livestock.
In Africa, the baobab is also used for worship and burial. The gigantic tree is at the heart of many proverbs, tales and epics. In fact, the first description of funeral customs in Senegal dates back to 1594. Until recent times, griots were buried in hollow baobabs. Burying griots, their wives and children, who are often despised and feared, in the open ground could spread disease and cause a lack of rain, making the soil, the cereals grown and the wells contaminated [7065] or the soil sterile for ever. Among the animist Sérères, the griot is mummified inside the baobab tree. His body is embalmed and dried inside. They were hung upright so that their bodies did not touch the ground, in order not to render it impure. This discriminatory practice was banned in 1962 by President Léopold Sédar Senghor. The same funeral practice is found in Burkina Faso, in the Dakoro region, and especially for lepers among all the Dogon of the plain. But it was the baobabs with a single upward opening that were favoured.
Still in Senegal, the baobab has a symbolic value in literary and artistic creations. A Wolof proverb says: *Ragal dou diam gouye* (The coward does not cut the baobab), because spirits can be disturbed and because he will not achieve his ends. And when it comes to respecting one's parents, the saying goes: *Lou gouye, réy réy gif a di ndeyam* (However great the baobab is, a simple seed is its mother). And among the Fon people of Benin, there's a saying about youthful ardour and pretensions: *Ab-dógbli ma zìn kpasa db* (Despite its power, the hand can never claim to topple a baobab)[66] .
Also in the Fon region of southern Benin, all baobabs are used as shelters for evil spirits and are therefore often mistrusted[67] . And along the Zambezi, some tribes believe that evil spirits bring misfortune to anyone who picks the tree's sweet white flowers. More specifically, a lion will kill them. Others believe that if you drink water containing baobab seeds, you will be safe from crocodile attacks. In Zambia, a baobab is said to be haunted by a ghostly python. Long

[65] "Le baobab en Afrique, plus qu'un symbole, une ressource : l'arbre aux mille usages", *Futura* , accessed 17/04/2024 (https://www.futura-sciences.com/planete/dossiers/botanique-baobab-arbre-pharmacien-arbre- vie-666/page/6/) p. 1-8.

[66] From our informant Daa Bokonon Segan, traditional doctor, diviner, priest of Fa (Bokonon) in Affossogba.

[67] Achille Ephrem Assogbadjo et als, "*Caractères morphologiques et production des capsules de baobab (Adansonia digitata L.) au Bénin", Fruits* 60/5 /09 (2005) p. 327-340.

ago, the python lived in the hollow trunk and was revered by the locals. A white hunter shot it, with bad consequences. Some nights, the locals can still hear the snake hissing.
In Zambia's Kafue National Park, one of the largest baobabs is known as *Kondanamwali*, or "the tree that eats young girls". The tree fell in love with four beautiful young girls. When they reached puberty, they made the tree jealous by finding husbands. Then, one night, during a storm, the tree opened its trunk and took the girls inside. A rest house was built in the branches of the tree. On stormy nights, the cries of the imprisoned girls can still be heard. Along the Limpopo River, it is believed that when a young boy bathes in the water used to soak baobab bark, he will become a great man. Others admit that women living in kraals where there are many baobabs will have more children. This is scientifically plausible, as these women have better access to the leaves and fruit, which are rich in vitamins and minerals.

4. Toxicity

Despite the many medicinal virtues that make the baobad an exceptional tree among plants, its careless use can cause problems. In fact, the powder can cause allergies, the main one being the appearance of certain gastric problems due to its high fibre content. To remedy this, simply reduce the dose. People with heart or kidney problems can potentially experience certain problems due to potassium. Furthermore, given that the fibre content per 100g of powder is 44g (i.e. around 10g more than the daily requirement for an adult), it is strongly recommended that people with intestinal problems avoid overdosing. As a precautionary measure, young children and pregnant or breast-feeding women should avoid taking baobab. People suffering from intestinal problems should take baobab with caution. Its high fibre content can cause bloating and flatulence. Taking baobab may cause side effects such as laxative effects, digestive discomfort, bloating and flatulence.

Baobab may contain potential anti-nutrients in its dried fruit pulp, such as cyanide and organic acids. However, these are below the detection level. Baobab seed oil may contain cyclopropane fatty acids, which can adversely affect fatty acid synthesis. However, its use has not shown any harmful effects in humans. This is because when the oils are cooked, the negative components are destroyed. It is clear that despite some scientific concerns about its consumption, baobab is in fact free from side effects and toxicity problems. Most studies have shown health benefits at a dose of 800 mg per kg of body weight for these anti-disease benefits. The ideal daily intake is probably around 23g of powder per day for optimum health[68] .

In the kitchen, with its tangy, slightly sweet taste, baobab powder can be combined with many different dishes and drinks: juices, smoothies, sorbets, ice creams, yoghurt, cereals, pancake mixes, cakes and cereal bars. Because of its sweet taste, it is possible to reduce the amount of sugar and flavour fromage frais, teas and infusions. And if you're feeling tired, it's advisable to take baobab powder as a cure at breakfast in drinks, cereals or other foods, while avoiding excessive consumption.

[68] Alice Pearson, "Baobab powder. Its multiple benefits", *Myprotein* (2017) p. 1-5.

CHAPTER 5

5. Outline of a botanical-morphological study of plants

To get a better idea of the richness of our investigations and to delve deeper into the therapeutic content of plants, it is important to draw up a morphological sketch of the plant. Each part, whether aerial, subterranean or aquatic, draws from its biological environment the substances necessary for photosynthesis, plant growth, inflorescence, fruit production, the formation of underground stems, rhizomes, bulbs and tubers, and the particular transformations of the root system. From the aerial apex to the root apex, all plant elements and their extracts are used in herbal remedies. Our methodology will consist of a five-stage presentation: stem, roots, leaves, flowers and fruits.

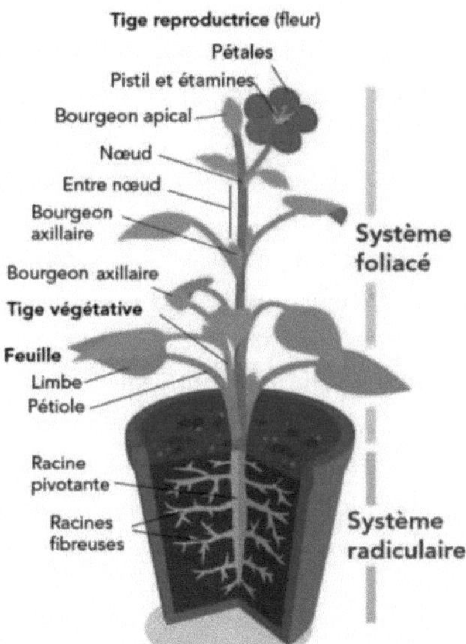

(Source: *Parlons Sciences*, 26/01/2023)[74]

5.1 The stem

The stem is the structure that forms the essential element of the root system. It is divided into two parts: the nodes and the internodes. The nodes are the places where buds appear and become leaves, other stems or flowers. The internodes are the parts of the stem between the nodes. The stem is the

[74] "The parts of a plant", Parlons Sciences 26/01 (2023) 1-3, Accessed 08/03/ 2024 (https://parlonssciences.ca/ressources-pedagogiques/documents-dinformation/les-parties-dune-plante).

The aerial part of a plant's anatomy that supports and structures it by supporting its other aerial plant organs, such as leaves and flowers. Another of its main characteristics is that it has negative geotropism, which means that it grows in the opposite direction to gravity.

Stems can be classified according to their growth medium. Aerial stems come in upright, creeping, climbing and voluble forms, or with spines, stolons or tendrils. The stems of most plants grow above ground, but the stems of some plants, such as potatoes, also grow below ground. The potato part is a specialised stem, called a tuber, which serves to store the plant's nutrients. The trunk is the name given to the stems of trees. The underground stems are subdivided into tubers, rhizomes and bulbs.

The role of the stem is to transport nutrients and substances within the plant. From the root, the so-called raw sap rises to the leaves through the canals of the stem, where it is enriched with carbon dioxide and gives rise to the elaborated sap. It supports the plant and enables the leaves, flowers and fruit to grow; it orientates the leaves towards the sun. It carries water and nutrients captured by the roots, as well as the products of photosynthesis carried out by the leaves.

There are four categories of aerial stems: the upright stem, which is sufficiently robust to grow vertically; the ascending stem, whose stock is perennial and robust but whose aerial stems are spindly and herbaceous; the lying or creeping stem, which is spread out on the ground and does not grow upwards or only slightly, it is also known as prostrate; the voluble stem, which surrounds a support in order to rest on it; the climbing stem, which attaches itself to a support by means of spikes, which are adventitious roots, or tendrils, which are transformed leaves. Aerial stems include cladodes, grass stubble, stipe (e.g. palms), cauline stems, succulent stems, stolons, root stems and specialised branches (spines, tendrils).

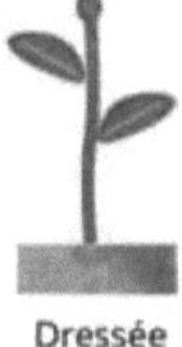

Dressée

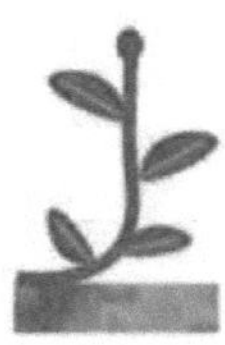

Montante

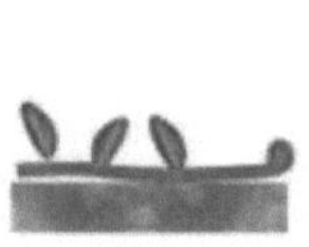

Couchée ou rampante

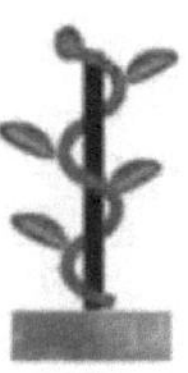

Volubile ou grimpante

The underground stems are: rhizomes that grow horizontally or obliquely in the soil. They bear roots or just a bunch of leaves; tubers, which develop in the soil, filling up with nutrients and bearing buds called "eyes"; bulbs, the short stem of which is called a plateau. At the top, they bear a terminal bud surrounded by leaves reduced to interlocking fleshy scales, gorged with nutrients.

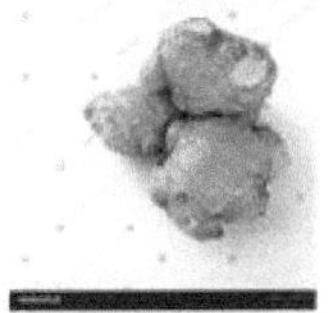

rhizome rhizome de gingembre

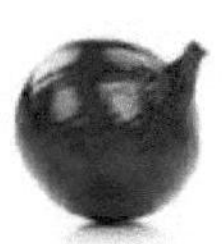

Bulbe d'oignon rouge

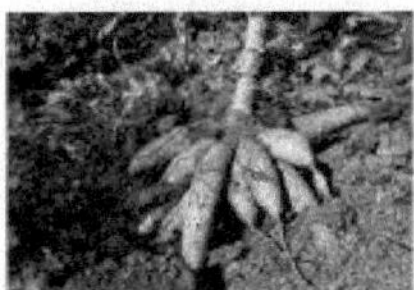

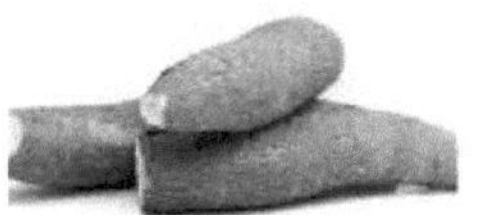

Tubercules de manioc

ginger rhizome red onion bulb
Cassava tubers

Aquatic stems that live submerged in water (hydrophytes). They are physiologically equipped to absorb water, carbon dioxide and oxygen directly, as well as nutrient salts. Plants such as *Ceratophyllum*, *Utricularia* and *Wolffia*, for example, do not have roots, which would be useless for nourishment. The cell wall of the epidermal cells on the stems of these plants is covered by a thin cuticle that is permeable to gases, water and solutes. Supporting tissues are not necessary because of buoyancy. On the other hand, most aquatic plants have a remarkable development of intercellular spaces which, by enclosing air, improve buoyancy and gas diffusion in the plant[72] (see aerenchyma).

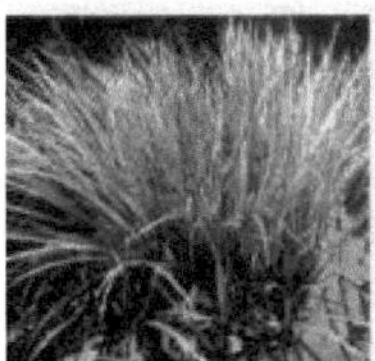
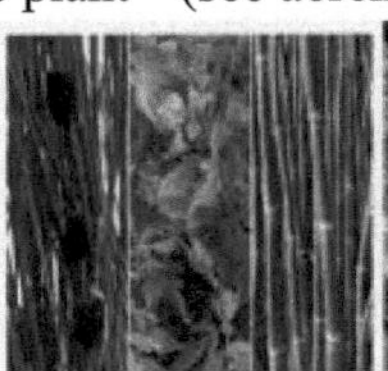
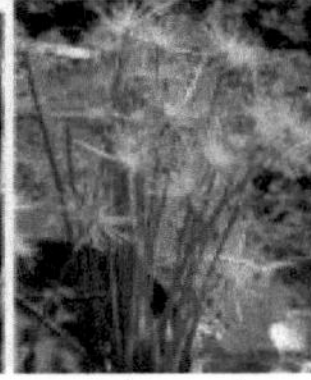

Sources: Tiges aquatiques, Accessed on 28/06/2023 (https://www.google.com/search?q=tiges+acquatiques&tbm=isch&ved=2ahUKEwis06H3meX)

[72] E. Strassburger, *Tratado de Botánica*, 8va. edición. Omega, Barcelona, 1994, 1088 p. (ISBN84-7102-990-1)

5.2 The roots

The root comes from the Low Latin *radicina, a* diminutive of the Latin *radix* (root, base, source, foundation) from which comes the Old French *rais* (root) which gives horseradish and radish. It is generally the underground organ of vascular plants, which attaches them to the soil and provides them with water and mineral salts. There are four types of root: stilt roots, which support the trunk above the ground or water (mangrove); aerial roots (epiphytic orchids); liana roots (banyan); sucker roots (vanilla). Their role is: to anchor the plant in the soil; to capture the water and minerals needed for plant growth; to store food and nutrients; to provide a means of reproduction called vegetative propagation (asexual). They generally find the little oxygen they need between grains of soil in the subsoil, but if the soil is saturated (full of water), the oxygen is driven out of the soil. If there is no oxygen below ground, plants will start to produce roots above ground. Roots can be thin and hair-like (fibrous roots) [A], short and thick (taproots) [B], or somewhere in between (e.g. anchor roots) [C].

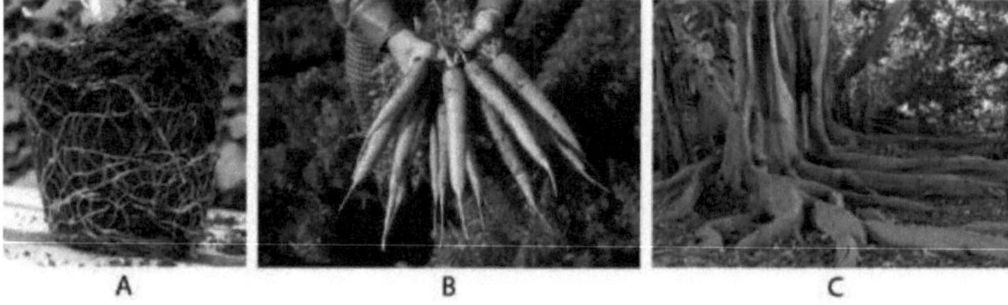

Fibrous roots of a tomato plant (A), taproots of carrot plants (B) anchoring roots of a fig tree (C) (Sources: (A) Rasbak at Dutch Wikipedia [CC BY-SA] via Wikimedia Commons; (B) Joe Larson / SDA Natural Resources Conservation Service [public domain] via Wikimedia Commons; (C) Patti Neumann [CC BY-SA] via Wikimedia Commons).

There are several types of root depending on the ecology of the plant. The taproot, which seeks water deep down. They are specific to trees and plants in dry regions. Fasciculated roots are roots that run below the surface of the soil. The adventitious root originates from a stem (underground or aerial) such as the stolons of a strawberry plant. They are often used for vegetative propagation and plant cuttings. The tracer root extends horizontally and can produce adventitious stems or suckers.

Since roots are the first organ that plants develop when they germinate, they can be distinguished by the anchorage they provide to the plant: contractile roots, stilt roots and epiphytic roots. Based on their shape, they can be classified as axonomorphic, fasciculated, napiform, branched or tuberous. They can also be classified according to the direction of growth as adventitious, aquatic, sucking, aerial and storage roots.

Their main function is to absorb water and nutrients through their small absorbent hairs, which they then pass on to the rest of the plant via the stem. They anchor the entire structure of the plant to the environment, either by underground roots that cling deeply, or by aerial roots that anchor themselves to other plants or surfaces. Some roots photosynthesise, or attach themselves to other plants to absorb nutrients.

It is important to note that in the case of taproots, the radicle sinks vertically and develops into a taproot (B). Frequently, the taproot system evolves, with adventitious roots emerging from the upper part of the taproot, which regresses, resulting in an adventitious root system (A). A taproot is a relatively straight, tapered plant root with positive orthogravitropism. It forms a pole from which other roots grow laterally. Plants with taproots are difficult to uproot and transplant. Their taproot system differs from the fasciculated and tracing root system.

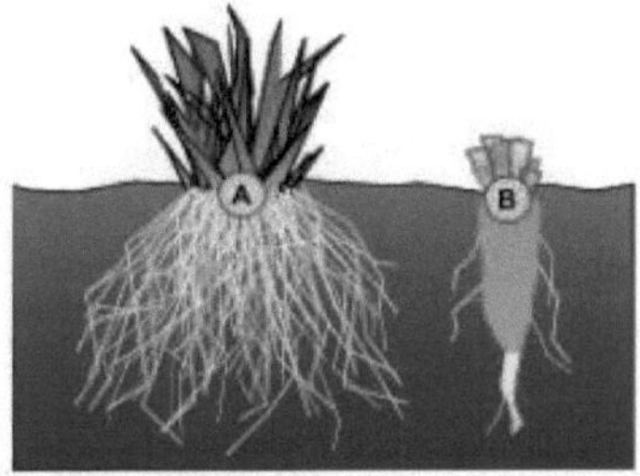

As for the shape of taproots, the following categories should be noted: the conical root, for example, the tuberised root of the carrot; the fusiform root, such as the radish root; and the napiform root, such as that of the turnip.

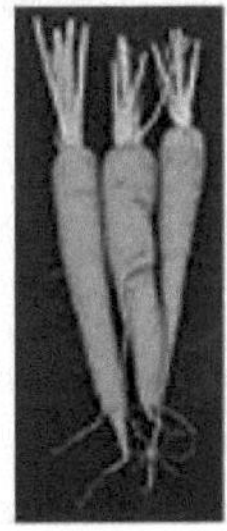
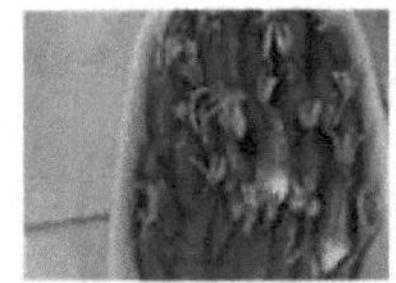
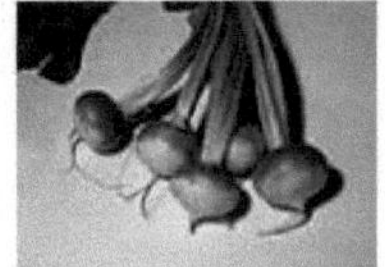

Conical root Fusiform root Napiform root

There are: tap roots or axonomorphs, fasciculated roots, napiform acines, branched acines and tuberous roots. But when it comes to roots according to the direction of growth, a distinction is made between: adventitious roots, aquatic roots, sucker roots, aerial acinar roots and storage roots. Then, when roots are considered in terms of anchorage, a distinction is made between: contractile roots, fulvic or stilt roots and epiphytic roots. The taproot or axonomorphic root is characterised by a main root, which is much thicker and larger, from which secondary roots of lesser length and thickness branch out.

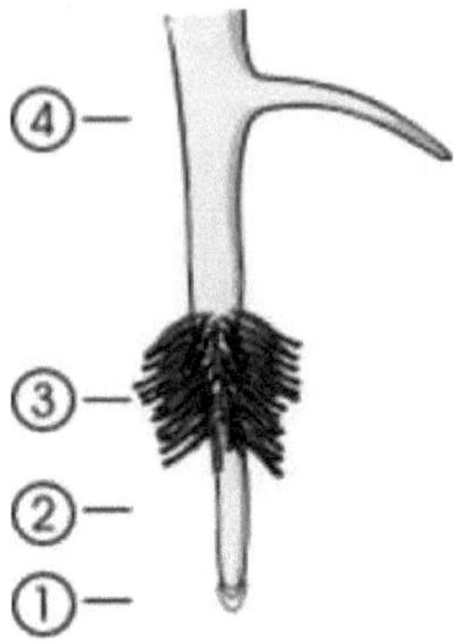

- The suberous zone (4) corresponds to the oldest part of the root; it bears the secondary roots or radicles.
- The piliferous zone (3) emits absorbent hairs. These absorb water and mineral salts.
- The growth zone (2) is located behind the cap and is responsible for cell multiplication.
- The cap (1) completes and protects the root. It is the cap that allows the root to penetrate the soil.

The facsiculated root, also known as the atypical or fibrous root, has no main root, so all the branches are of equal importance and can reach similar sizes. This is one of the most common types found in garden plants.

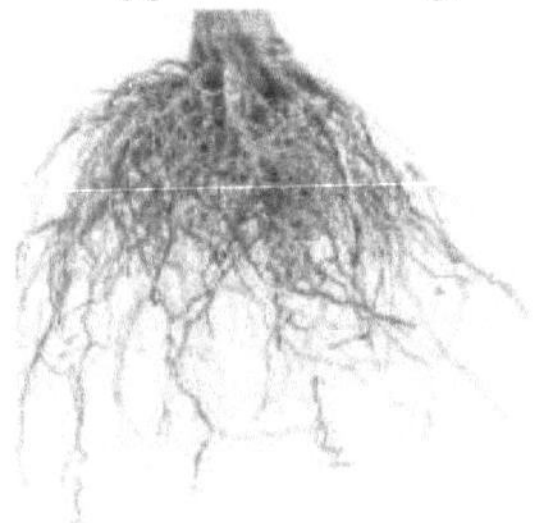

In the case of nappiform roots, the plant contains a large main root that has evolved to store reserves of nutrients and other vital substances. These are very thick roots, many of which are edible.

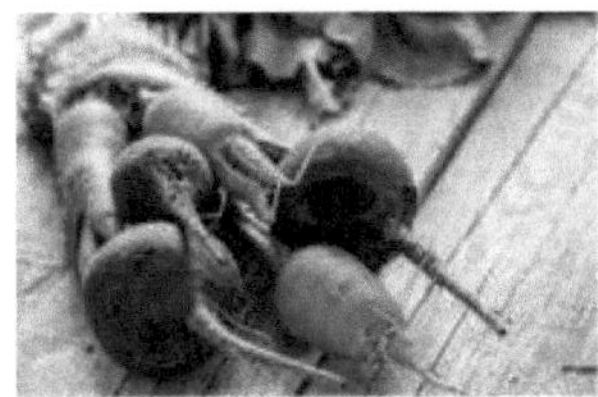

Nappiform roots

The structure of the branched root is reminiscent of the branches of a tree. It has no main root and branches out in a very pronounced way.

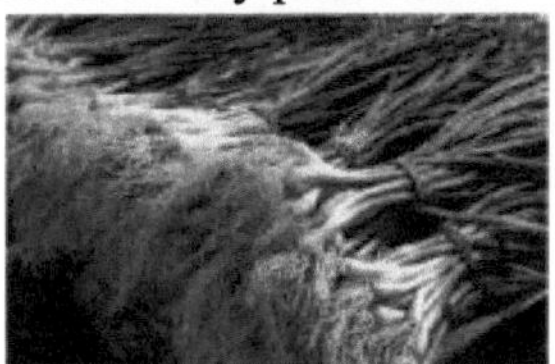

Branched root

Tuberous roots also have the capacity to develop and grow by storing reserve substances. This can occur in several roots, not just the main one. They are generally confused as tubers.

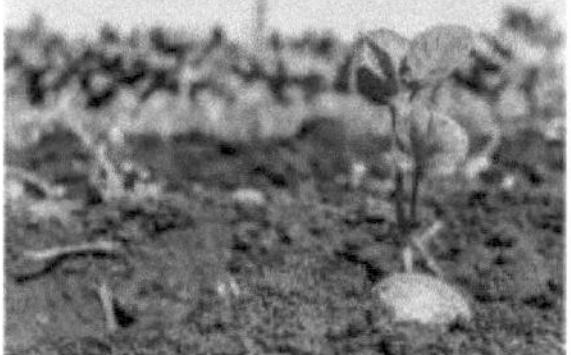

Tuberous root

Adventitious roots are roots that grow above the soil. They remain in contact with the soil in order to absorb nutrients and water, but grow above it without burying themselves. These roots are subdivided into the following categories: foliar, fibrous and adventitious.

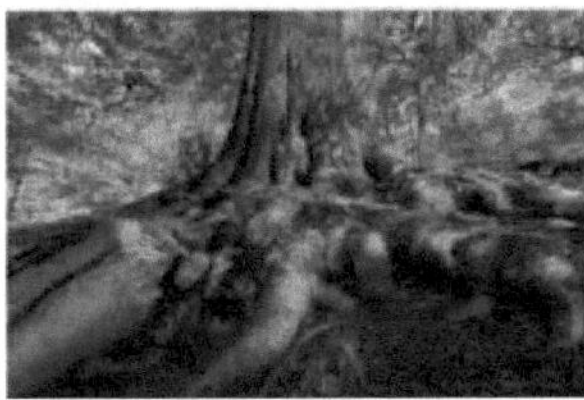

Adventitious root

Aquatic roots are characteristic of aquatic plants. They are not in contact with the ground and draw the nutrients needed by plants that grow in aquatic environments. Generally, these are plants that are not attached to surfaces and simply float on water.

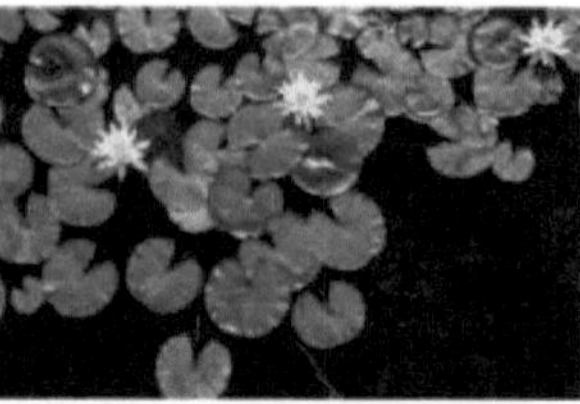

Aquatic root

Parasitic plants can develop roots that penetrate the branches or stems of the plants they parasitise, absorbing the nutrients they need. These are called suckers or parasitic roots.

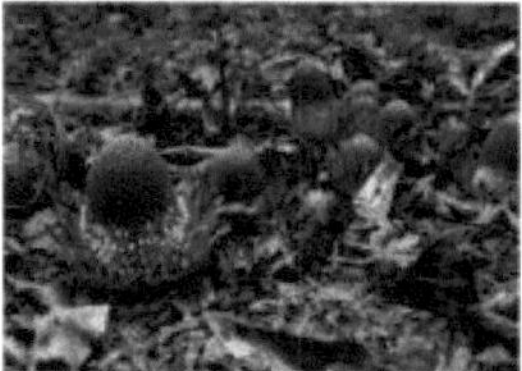

Parasitic or "sucker" root

Aerial roots are parasitic plants which grow their roots downwards and can strangle the host plant.

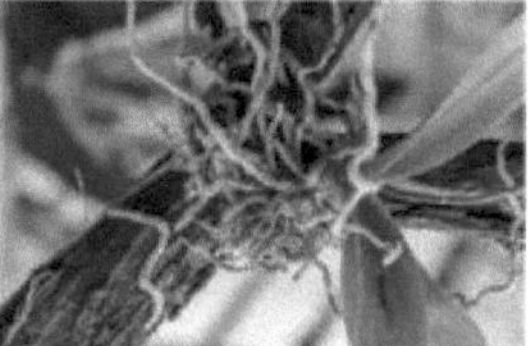

Aerial root

Storage roots belong to the category of tubers and other roots that are capable of storing water and nutrients underground, in order to protect them from herbivorous predators and to be able to use them according to the plant's needs.

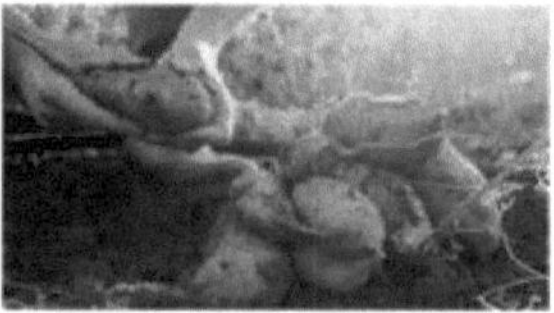

Storage root

Contractile roots are also a type of adventive root. They are roots whose function is to move the shoot to a location close to the soil surface. Contractile roots are long and fleshy, part of which is consumed as the plant grows.

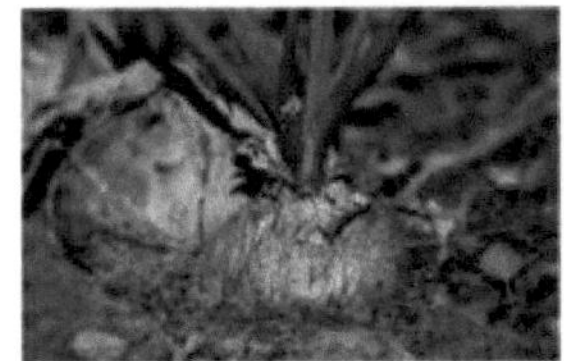

Contractile root

Fluvial roots or stilt roots. These roots start at the base of the trunk or stem before reaching the ground. From there, they grow and extend into the ground, even passing through water, so that part of them remains visible. They are generally found in large trees, which require greater stability due to the environment in which they grow.

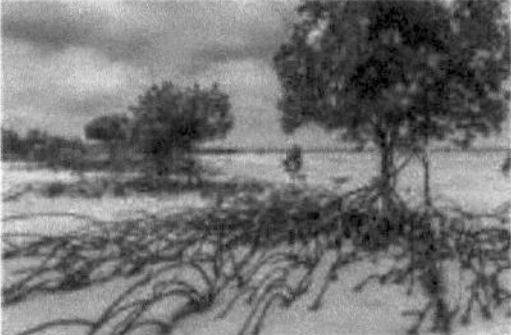

River root

Epiphytic roots are developed by plants that grow on the surface of other plants but do not parasitise them. They do not absorb nutrients from the supporting plant, but simply anchor themselves to it.

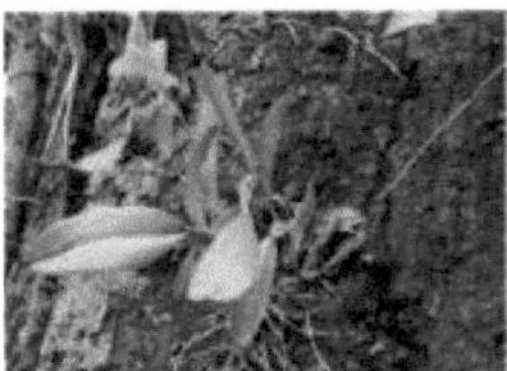

Epiphytic root

Edible roots include ginger, turmeric, yucca, beetroot, potato, carrot, liquorice, parsnip, radish, valerian, ginseng, manioc, yam, potato and taro. These species are generally rich in carbohydrates and starch. Wild edible species include: Mandil - Trifolium alpinum, Wild garlic - Allium vineale, Wild carrot - Daucus carota.

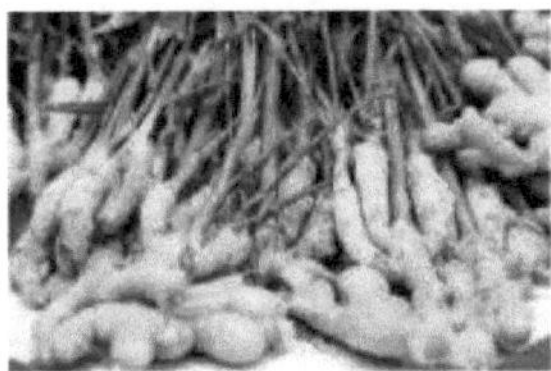

Edible roots

5.3 Leaves

The leaf is the organ specialising in photosynthesis in vascular plants, inserted into plant stems at the nodes. It is also the site of respiration and transpiration. They can specialise, in particular to store nutrients and water. They generally consist of a flat, thin aerial blade, the limbus, which allows the maximum surface area to be exposed to light. On the other hand, other leaves with a very reduced blade no longer play a photosynthetic role. They are transformed into tendrils, cataphylls, scales on buds, aerial (spines, conifer needles) or underground (as in bulbs, corms), succulent leaves. It is the palisade parenchyma, a particular type of leaf tissue, which carries out photosynthesis thanks to its cells containing chloroplasts, and gives the leaf its green colour. Foliage or foliage is an uncountable name that designates, for annual plants, the appearance of leaves, a seasonal phase concomitant with budburst. The leaves of some vegetables, such as turnips, are called "tops"; other edible leaves are called "brèdes".

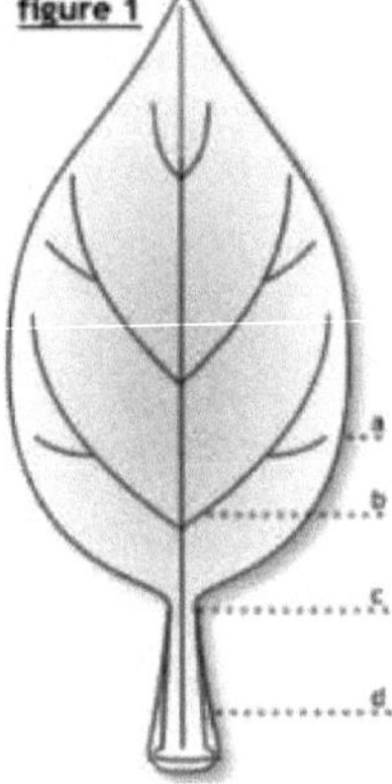

The different parts of the leaf: a flat blade (a) with veins (b), often with a petiole (c) which attaches the leaf to the stem, sometimes enlarged into a sheath (d). This may "embrace" the stem, as in the Poaceae. The petiole may be absent, in which case the leaf is said to be sessile. It may sometimes be winged, or have more or less developed stipules at its base. At the point of insertion of the petiole and the stem, there is an axillary bud.
Source: https://fr.wikipedia.org/wiki/Feuille.

The auxiliary bud is at the point of insertion of the leaf on the stem and will give rise to a new shoot or flower. The leaf blade is furrowed with veins that form a vascular network through which the sap circulates. The main (or mid) vein is followed by the secondary veins and, eventually, the veins. On the upper surface, the veins are generally recessed, whereas on the lower surface they are more prominent.

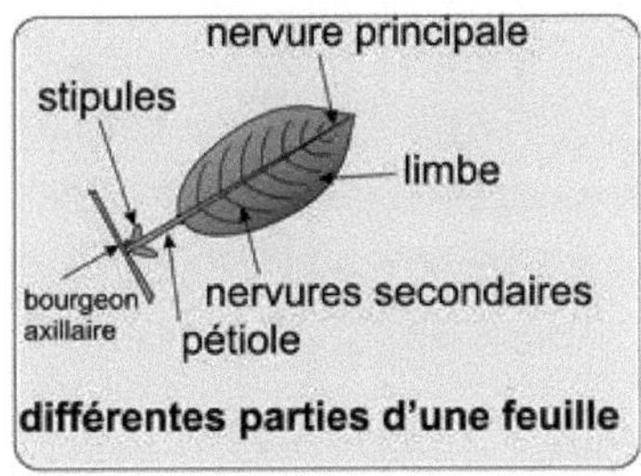

Source[76] :[78]

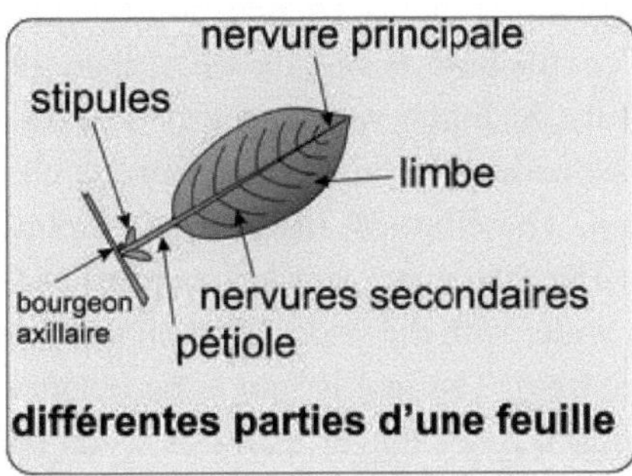

Different parts of a leaf

Simple leaves have a single, continuous blade, whereas compound leaves are made up of several leaflets attached to the petiole by petioles . Leaflets are not leaves, but parts of a single leaf.

The leaflets are never attached to the stem, but to the petiole, and they never have an axillary bud.

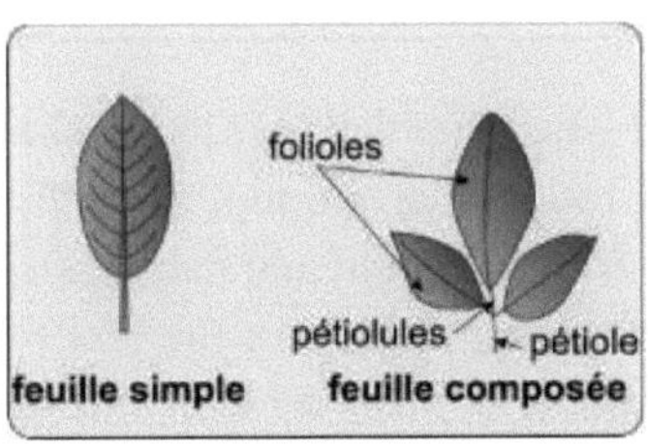

The leaves can be distinguished by their shape: whole, oval, obovate, elliptical, lanceolate, oblanceolate.

[78] "La feuille, description globale", Les Jardins du Gué 27/12 (2010), consulted on 25/06/2023 (https://www.jardinsdugue.eu/la-feuille-description-globale/)

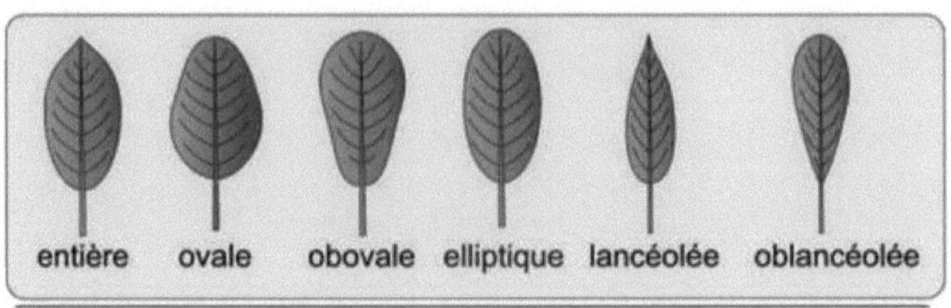

The whole leaf is the leaf blade, which has no divisions, teeth or cut-outs and no protrusions, like the laurel and cherry (*Prunus laurocerasus*). The oval leaf has an egg-shaped blade, i.e. the base is slightly wider than the top, like *Hypericum androsaemum* (one of the St John's wort species). The obovate leaf is also egg-shaped, but this time the widest part is at the top (prefix ob = upside down), as in *Arctostaphylos uva-ursi*. The elliptical leaf has an elliptical blade, like the leaf of *Asclepias cornutii.* The lanceolate leaf has a spearhead-shaped blade, 3 to 4 times longer than it is wide, with the widest part on the petiole side, like the leaf of *Olea europea* (olive tree). The leaf is said to be oblanceolate when the blade is spearhead-shaped, 3 to 4 times longer than it is wide, but the widest part is at the top and not at the base like the leaf of *Daphne mezereum.*

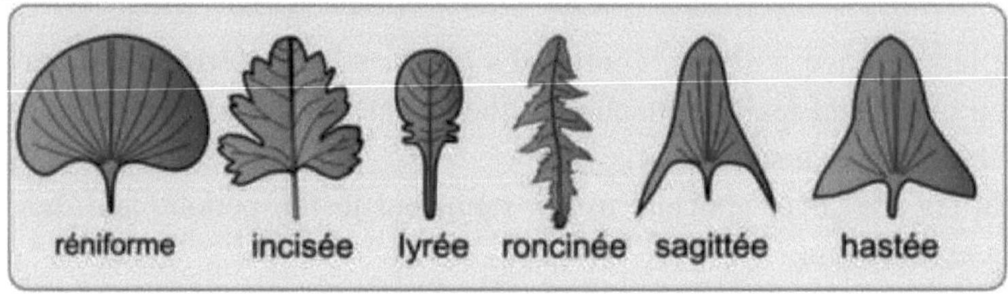

The leaf is kidney-shaped when the blade is kidney-shaped, wider than it is long, indented at the base and rounded at the top, as in *Farfugium japonicum.* It is incised when the blade is irregularly cut and the incisions are deeper than simple teeth, but do not reach the main vein, as in the leaf of *Veronica austriaca ssp. Teucrium.* The leaf is lyrate or lyriform when the upper lobe is much larger and rounded above the much smaller lower lobes, as in the rutabaga leaf. It is said to be stalked when the blade has deep, acute teeth that are turned down towards the base, as in the case of the dandelion leaf (*Taraxacum dens-leonis).* When the blade is arrowhead-shaped, the leaf is said to be sagittate, like that of *Arisarum vulgare.* But when the blade is halberd-shaped, with the two lobes at the base almost horizontal, unlike a sagittate leaf, it is called a hastate leaf, like the leaf of *Atriplex hastata*.

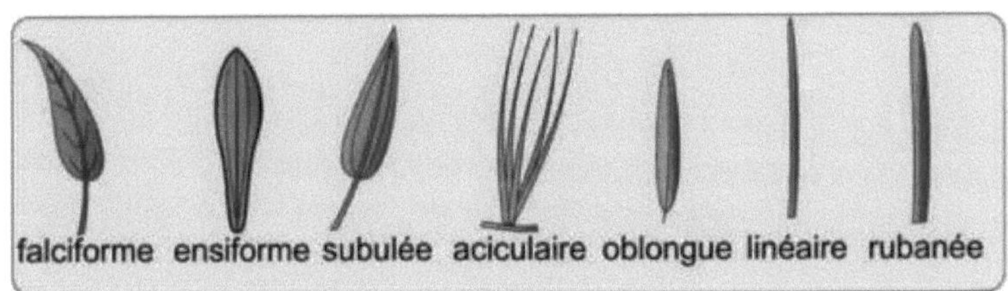

The leaf is said to be falcate or falcate when the blade is shaped like a scythe or sickle. This is the case with the leaf of *Iris acutiloba.* the central vein than at the edges, like the leaf of *Eryngium yuccifolium.* But when the blade is shaped like a cobbler's awl, with rather parallel edges and ending in a point, it is said to be subulate, like that of *Sagina subulata.* And when the blade is needle-shaped (from the Latin "acicula" =needle), elongated, thin and ending in a point, the leaf is said to be acicular or aculeate, like that of conifer needles. It is said to be oblong when the blade is clearly longer than it is wide, with almost parallel margins, like that of *Aster lateriflorus.* However, when the leaf blade is very long and narrow, with parallel edges, it is called a linear leaf, like that of the carnation (*Dianthus*). And when the blade is ribbon-shaped and the two ends are roughly equal in width, the leaf is said to be ribboned, like that of *Clivia nobilis.*

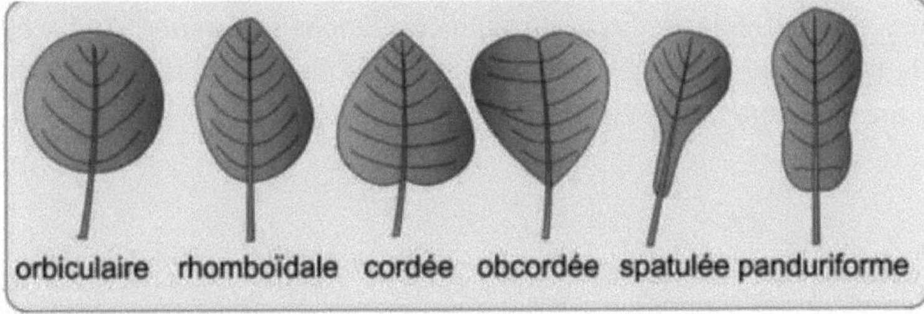

When the leaf is orbicular (from the Latin "orbis" = sphere), the blade is almost circular in shape. This is the case with the leaf of *Cercis chinensis.* And when the blade is diamond-shaped, the leaf is said to be rhomboidal or rhombic or rhomboid (from the Greek *rhombos*: spinning top, diamond). This is the case for the leaf of *Cissus rhombifolia.* The leaf is cordate or cordate-shaped when the blade is heart-shaped, like that of *Peperomia marmorata.* It is also said to be obcordate when the blade is heart-shaped, but with the point at the bottom, in contrast to cordate leaves. This is the case with the leaf of *Oxalis stricta.* The leaf is spatulate when the blade is spatula-shaped, broad at the top and narrow and elongated at the base, as in the leaf of *Primula frondosa.* And when the blade is constricted in the middle or lower part, a bit like a figure eight or a violin, the leaf is said to be panduforme. This is the case with *Rumex pulcher.*

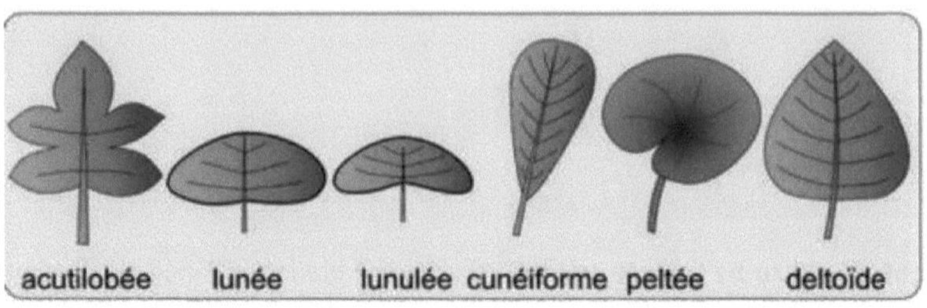

The leaf is said to be acutilobate when the lobes of the blade are pointed or even prickly, as in the case of the leaf of *Hepatica acutiloba.* It is lunate when the blade is shaped like a half-moon. This shape, as well as the following one, applies in particular to fern pinnae, i.e. the small subdivisions of fern fronds. When the leaf blade is in the shape of a crescent moon, smaller than that of a lunate leaf, it is called a lunulate leaf. On the other hand, it is said to be wedge-shaped or cuneate when the blade is in the shape of an inverted wedge or triangle, i.e. with the point at the bottom. This is the case with the leaf of *Echeveria ciliata.* A peltate leaf is one in which the petiole is not attached to the base of the blade but practically in the centre of its surface, which is generally orbicular. An example is the nasturtium *leafTropaelum majus.* And when the blade is triangular, like the Greek capital *delta*, the leaf is said to be **deltoid**. This is the case with the leaf of *Populus deltoides.*

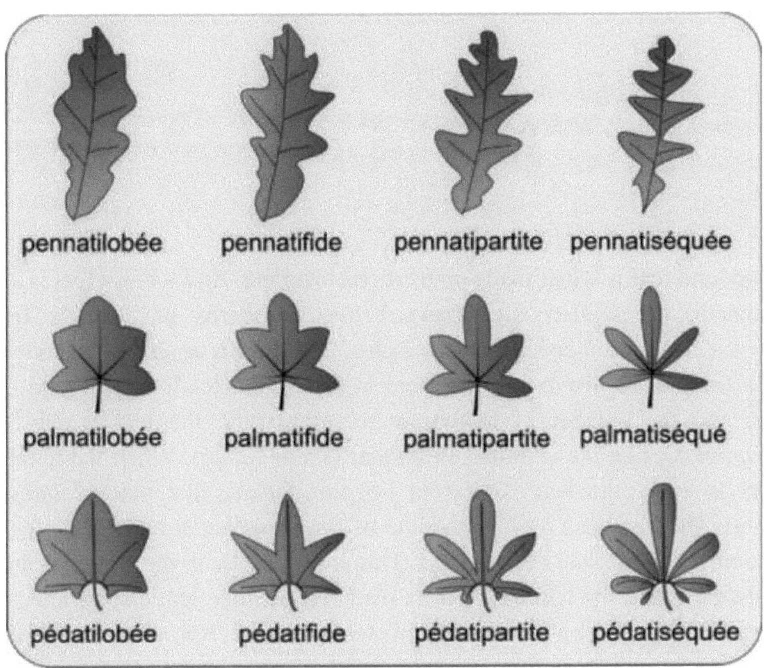

Here, we need to consider both the network of veins and the depth of the indentations in the leaf blade. The veins are said to be ***pinnate*** when they are arranged like the barbs of a bird's feathers or the teeth of a comb, as on a pear leaf. They are *palmate* when they all start at the same point at the base of the leaf and spread out like the fingers of a hand, like a vine leaf. They are said to be *pedate* or *pedalled* when the base of the leaf blade has two very divergent main veins which bear secondary veins perpendicular to the main veins on their inner side only, as on a hellebore leaf. With regard to the depth of the indentations, and applying this first to pinnately venationed leaves: when the indentations are shallow, the leaf blade is *pennatilobed.* When the indentations reach about the middle of each half-blade, the leaf is said to be *pennatifid* (Latin *fidus*, split). When the notches reach beyond the middle of the half-blade without reaching the main blade, the leaf is said to be *pennatipartite* (Latin *partitus*, divided). Then, when the notches reach the main vein, the leaf is said to be *pennatipartite* (Latin *sectus*, cut). The same logic applied to palmately venationed leaves will give the following terms: *palmatilobed, palmatifid, palmatipartite* and *palmatiséquée*. And for leaves with pedate venation, we have *pedatilobed, pedatifid*, *pedatipartite* and *pedatisse* leaves.

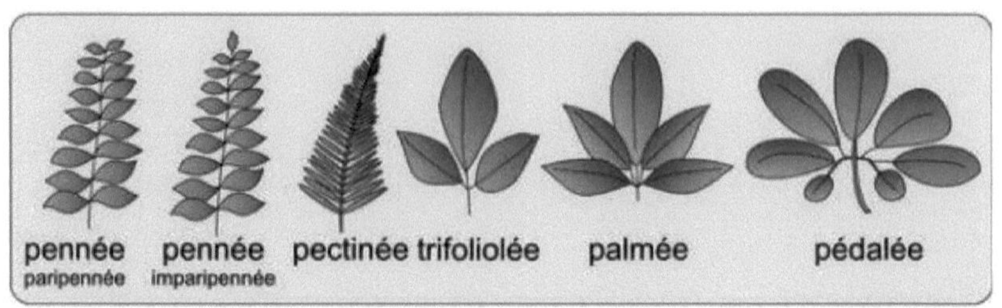

A compound leaf is a leaf made up of several leaflets. And when a leaf is said to be pinnate, the leaflets are arranged like the barbs of a bird's feather, symmetrically on either side of the rachis. The ***rachis is*** the extension of the petiole for pinnate leaves. When there is a terminal leaflet at the end of the rachis, and the number of leaflets is therefore odd, the leaf is said to be *imparipinnate*, like the common vetch leaf (*Vicia sativa*). When the number of leaflets is even, the leaf is said to be *paripinnate*, like that of *Indigofera tinctoria.* The *pectinate leaf* is made up of fine lamellae arranged like the teeth of a comb on either side of the rachis. This is the case with the leaves of the yew tree (*Taxus*). And the trifoliate leaf is made up of three leaflets, all attached to the top of the petiole, as in the leaf of *Acer griseum.* NB: the term trifoliolate should be distinguished from ***ternate***, which means arranged in threes. Thus, three leaves starting from the same point are said to be ternate, not trifoliate, because they are not leaflets. There are also ***biternate*** (twice ternate) and ***triternate*** (three times ternate) arrangements. The leaf is said to be palmate when there are more than 3 leaflets attached to the top of the petiole and fanning out; this is called a palmate leaf, as in the horse chestnut *Aesculus californica.* The pedalled leaf is made up of leaflets arranged as if attached to the petiole of the preceding leaflet, like the hellebore leaf (*Helleborus viridis).*

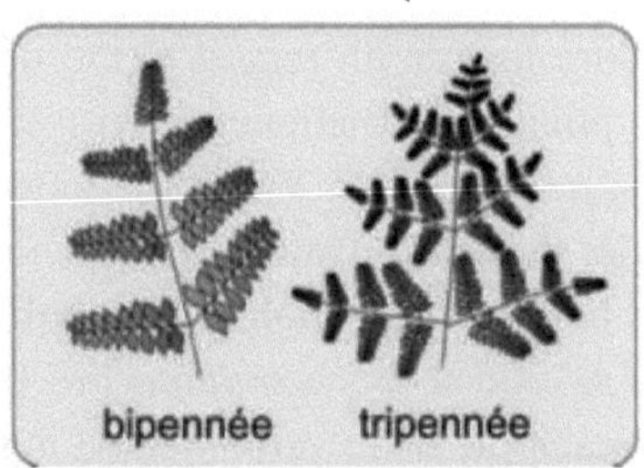

On the subject of pinnate leaves, if the leaflets themselves are pinnate, the leaf is said to be ***bipinnate***. And if the second level leaflets are also pinnate, the leaf is said to be ***tripinnate.*** Ferns even have ***quadripinnate*** leaves.

Leaves have three main functions. They carry out photosynthesis, obtaining chemical energy from the sun's rays. They allow the plant to breathe, exchanging gases at night. They can even transpire, allowing excess water to escape through them. Leaves are the flattened green parts of plants called limbs. They are attached to the stem by the petiole. Most leaves have these parts, but not all. Leaves are usually broad and flat to expose their chloroplasts to as much sunlight as possible. The needles of pine and other conifers are leaves. Their small surface area combined with a waxy coating minimises water loss.

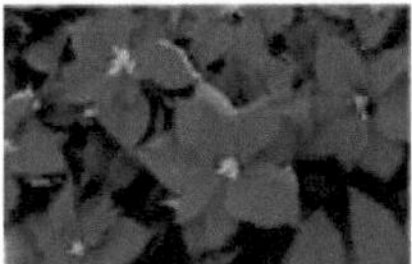

The red bracts of a poinsettia[77]

In short, the primary function of leaves is chlorophyll photosynthesis, which takes place in three stages: the use of light through the leaf blade as an efficient solar collector; the exchange of gases (CO_2, O2 and evaporation of H_2O); and the transport of raw and processed sap via a very extensive network of veins. Leaves can also absorb nutrients other than CO_2. This transfer, which seems to take place slowly through the cuticle and/or more rapidly via the stomata, is sometimes a determining factor in the transfer of metals from the air to the plant. Leaf morphology is one of the factors that may or may not favour the deposition and subsequent adsorption or absorption and internalisation of atmospheric particles. This can pose environmental health problems, for example when it concerns vegetables or other crops for human or animal consumption (fodder, etc.), especially if the toxic substance is mainly stored in the edible parts (leaves, fruit, seeds, tubers). Leaves also play a part in defending plants against herbivores by synthesising tannins, alkaloids or PR proteins, and protecting foliage against photo-oxidation.

[77] What look like large red flowers are in fact specialised structures called bracts. These are specialised leaves whose role is to attract pollinators such as bees and birds. The flowers are the small yellow structures in the centre of the bracts. Many flowers are attractive to animals such as birds and bees, which carry the pollen (which contains the male reproductive cells) from one flower to another. These animals are called pollinators because they help to distribute the pollen.

In aquatic environments, the leaves absorb nutrients dissolved in the water, sometimes more than the roots, which are mainly used for anchoring. Thorny plants often transform their leaves into spines by modifying the leaflets, stipules or simply the hairs. Like xerophilous plants, this is a defence mechanism against drought, or against grazing by herbivorous animals. Some very fine spines and cilia enable the plant to collect dew. Carnivorous plants take on highly specialised forms, such as the *urn* shape of Nepenthes or the trap shape of

Dionaea, which have a leaf blade in two parts fitted with prickles and capable of folding over each other to trap insects. The leaves of succulents and succulent plants are often transformed into reserve organs. The leaves or leaflets of climbing plants are transformed into tendrils enabling them to cling to their support. This role is sometimes played by the petiole. Aquatic plants, such as the water hyacinth, can transform their leaves into tendrils. The leaves of plants adapted to drought (xerophilous) can be reduced to scales (they are called "squamiform") or needles (conifers). The plant reduces its leaf area in order to limit evapotranspiration. The holm oak, for example, can have several leaf shapes: in a favourable environment, where air humidity is not limiting, it will have leaves with an almost oval blade, whereas in a dry environment, the leaves will be mostly toothed. Some species of epiphytes, such as the Bromeliads, use their leaves to collect and store water.

5.4 The flower

The flower is a stem of limited growth that develops modified leaves at its tip, which have a reproductive function. These structures are called anthophylls (these are the petals and sepals) and have different parts, each specialising in one or more functions, such as gamete formation, fruit and seed dispersal, pollination and other protective structures.

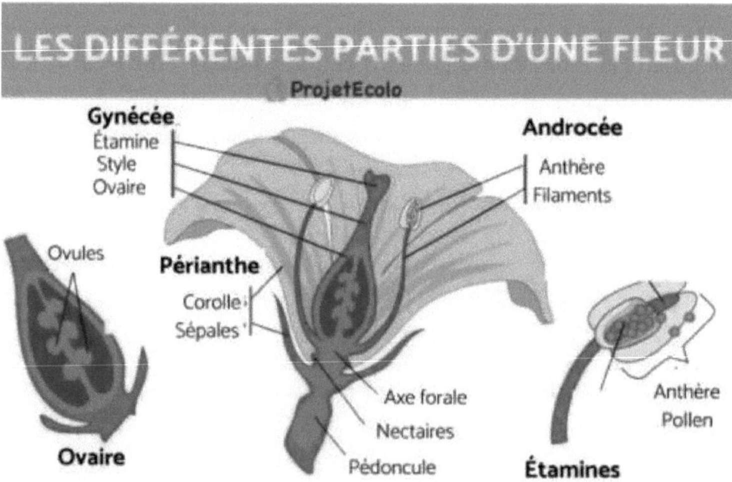

Source[78] :

Spermatophytes or phanerogams are seed-producing plants whose flowers are the part of the plant that houses the reproductive structures[79] . Thus, in the flowers, the gametes

78
Antoine Decrouy, "Composition of a flower - the different parts of a flower", Projet Ecolo 12/05
(2023) 1-3 , Accessed on 25/06/2023 (https://www.projetecolo.com/composition-d-une-fleur-les-differentes- parties-d-une-fleur-192.html).

79 The part of the flower that does not have a reproductive function is called the perianth and is formed by the calyx made up of sterile structures: the sepals, the corolla, formed by the petals. The parts of a flower with reproductive functions are: the androecium, formed by the stamens with their pollen grains (male reproductive organs), the gynoecium, formed by the pistils with their carpels (male and female reproductive organs, part of the flower where fertilisation takes place and where the seeds are created. They also have structures for protection and germination. The flowers are responsible for the plant's reproduction. This is why they are often brightly coloured to attract pollinating insects. But not all plants reproduce through flowers. They come in many shapes and sizes, colours, forms and fragrances. The flower has **a calyx, a corolla, stamens, a filament and pistils.** In the stamens, the plant's male sexual organ, is the pollen which, when transported to the pistils, the female sexual organ, gives rise to the process of creating a new plant.

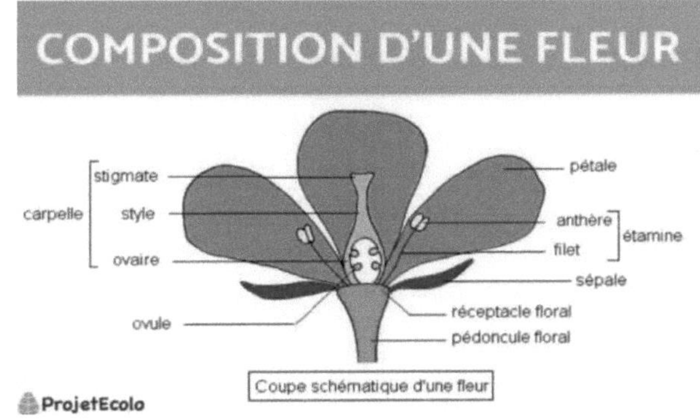

Source[80]

females), the carpels, which are further divided into ovary, style and stigma.

80 Antoine Decrouy, "Composition d'une fleur - Les différentes parties d'une fleur", *Projet Ecolo* 12/05 (2023) 1-3 , consulted on 25/06/2023 (https://www.projetecolo.com/composition-d-une-fleur-les- differentes-parties-d-une-fleur-192.html).

The different parts of the flower have different functions. The peduncle: this is the stem that supports the flower. It does not form part of the floral parts; the floral receptacle or thalamus which is an enlargement of the peduncle where the anthophylls or floral parts are inserted. The calyx is the part of the flower made up of leaf-like structures, usually green, called sepals. The function of the calyx is to protect the flower bud; the corolla is the part of the flower formed by leaf-like structures, usually coloured and called petals. The petals are formed after the sepals and their function is to be pollinated; to do this, they use their shapes and bright colours to attract pollinators; the androecium is the part of the flower containing the male reproductive organs: the stamens. In the male part of the flower, each stamen consists of a filament at the end of which it widens to form the anther, where the male gametes or pollen grains, also known as microgametophytes, are produced; the *gynoecium* is the part of the flower containing the female reproductive organs. This female part of the flower is formed by the pistil, which in turn is formed by the carpels. A carpel is divided into three parts. The ovary, which is the enlarged part containing the ovule. The style is the elongated area between the ovary and the stigma. And finally, the stigma, which is the final part of the style and is a sticky structure, since its function is to capture the pollen grains.

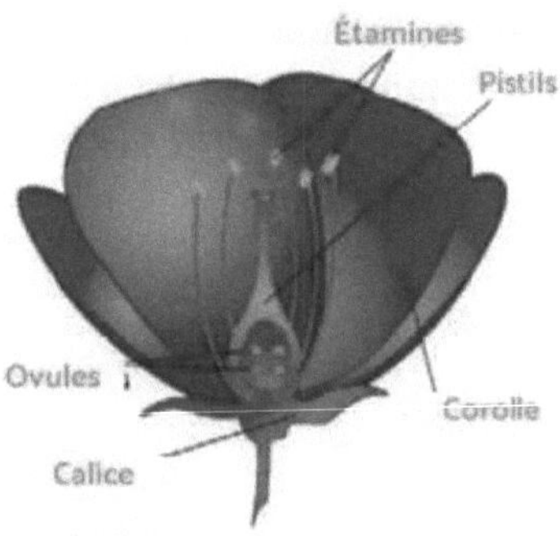

There are different varieties of flowers. The flowers of angiosperm plants, which are the typical flowers, can be classified from different points of view. If we classify angiosperm flowers according to their reproductive part, we differentiate between species with male flowers (only stamens), female flowers (only pistils) and hermaphrodite flowers (both types of reproductive organs). If we classify them according to the presence of all the floral structures (sepals, petals, stamens and pistil), we divide them into two categories: complete flowers, which have all four elements of a typical flower. A typical example is the rose. These are hermaphrodite flowers; incomplete flowers do not have all four elements. An example is the begonia, which is made up of stamens or pistils, but never both. They correspond to flowers that have only one sex. Another way of classifying them is to take into account the number of cotyledons in which the seed develops. A distinction is made between: monocotyledons, in which the flower develops on a single cotyledon supplied by the seed. Their leaves have a single parallel vein. Examples of this type of flower include lilies, orchids, tulips, crocuses, daffodils and campanulas;

dicotyledons, where the flower develops on two single cotyledons supplied by the seed. Their veins start at the bottom and branch out towards the surface, like roses, daisies, nasturtiums and begonias.

Let's take the example of the maize inflorescence. This is a monoecious plant, with unisexual flowers (i.e. separate male and female flowers on the same plant). The male inflorescence is called the panicle and the female inflorescence is called the ear. The spike is covered with specialised leaves called spathes. At floral induction[79] , the apical meristem of the stem becomes an apical inflorescence meristem which produces the panicle[80] . Formation of the panicle begins when the apical inflorescence meristem produces a series of lateral meristems; the first of these are called shoot meristems and are responsible for forming the main branches of the panicle[81] . The next lateral meristems (further away from the vegetative stem) develop spikelet pair meristems, which may form on the meristems of the branches[82] . Each spikelet pair meristem produces a small shoot with 2 spikelet meristems, each of which produces a primordial glume and develops 2 floral meristems (upper and lower). Each floral meristem produces the floral organs (the palea, two glumellae, three stamens and a pistil) and is supported by the lemma. Pistil development is arrested, resulting in the formation of a unisexual male inflorescence. Most of the auxiliary meristems remain dormant. However, some of the lower meristems can generate tillers and some of the upper meristems can generate spikes[83] . Spikes are formed from auxiliary meristems that have become inflorescence meristems and then developed into spikes through a reiterative process of meristem formation and organ differentiation[84] . Each spikelet pair meristem will trigger the formation of a spikelet meristem and will itself become a spikelet meristem. Each spikelet meristem then triggers the formation of a floral meristem, which in turn becomes a floral meristem. The duration and intensity of this repetitive process of spikelet pair meristem formation determines the number of floras in the formation of the adult spike. Some observations suggest that genotypes that

79 The transition from vegetative to reproductive growth.

80 Jackson, S.D, "Plant responses to photoperiod". *The New Phytologist* 181 (2009) p. 517-531.

81 Colasanti J. et al, *The maize floral transition. Bennetzen JL*, (2009) (eds) Handbook of Maize: Its Biology, Springer, New York, USA, p 41-55.

82 M. J. T Norman et als, *The ecology of tropical food crops*. Cambridge University Press (1995).

83 C. W. Smith et als, *Corn: Origin, history, technology, and production*. John Wiley & Sons (2004).

84 P. McSteen et als, "A floret by any other name: control of meristem identity in maize", *Trends in Plant Science* 5 (2000) p. 61-66.

produce inflorescences later develop more florules per row[85] . Each inflorescence is surrounded by modified leaves that act as protective envelopes (i.e. spathes)[86] . The spikes form bristles from their ovules. Silk development begins at the base of the spike and continues towards the top over the course of several days. Normally, the release of pollen and the appearance of silks are synchronous, resulting in high grain production. However, severe stresses such as drought can delay silk emergence and reduce pollen grain production[87] . The delay between pollen release and silk emergence is known as the anthesis-flowering interval[88] . Pollen is released continuously for a week or more; a release of around 10 million pollen grains for each maize panicle[89] . Pollen can be released easily (e.g. in response to vibrations or light winds) and dispersed over short distances of up to 30 m[90] . The viability of the pollen decreases once it is released from the panicle[91] . In some cases, horizontal winds allow pollen to travel several hundred metres[92] . The pollen grains fall from the panicle (known as anthesis) onto the spike bristles, which are covered in sticky hairs that capture the pollen grains[93] . The pollen grains germinate immediately and a pollen tube is inserted into the silk, transferring the genetic material to the female ovule and causing fertilisation.

---

85 R.M. Bonhomme et als, "Flowering of diverse maize cultivars in relation to temperature and
photoperiod in multilocation field trials", *Crop Science* 34 (1994) p. 156-164.

86 B. G. Cook et als, "Tropical Forages: an interactive selection tool", Accessed on 24/08/2023 (https://www.tropicalforages.info/text/intro/index.html) p. 1.

87 A.J. Hall et als, "Water stress before and during flowering in maize and its effects on yield, its components, and their determinants", *Maydica 26* (1981) p. 26:19-38.

88 J. Bolaños et al, "The importance of the anthesis-silking interval in breeding for drought tolerance in tropical maize", *Field Crops Research* 48 (1996) p. 65-.

89 M.Bannert et al, "Cross-pollination of maize at long distance", *European Journal of Agronomy* 27/1 (2007) p. 44-51.

90 D.E. Aylor, "Rate of dehydration of corn (*Zea mays*) pollen in the air". *Journal of Experimental Biology* 54/391 (2003) p. 2307-2312.

91 E. H. Coe et als, "The genetics of corn. (1988) p. 81-257 *in* F. Sprague, J. W. Dudley, eds. Corn and Corn Improvement (Third Edition), Madison, Wisconsin, USA.

92 D.E. Aylor, 2003. "Rate of dehydration of corn (*Zea mays*) pollen in the air". *Journal of Experimental Biology* 54/391 (2003) p. 2307-2312.

93 *A. S Hitchcock,. 1971, Manual of the grasses of the United States. Courier Corporation, US Department of Agriculture* (1971).

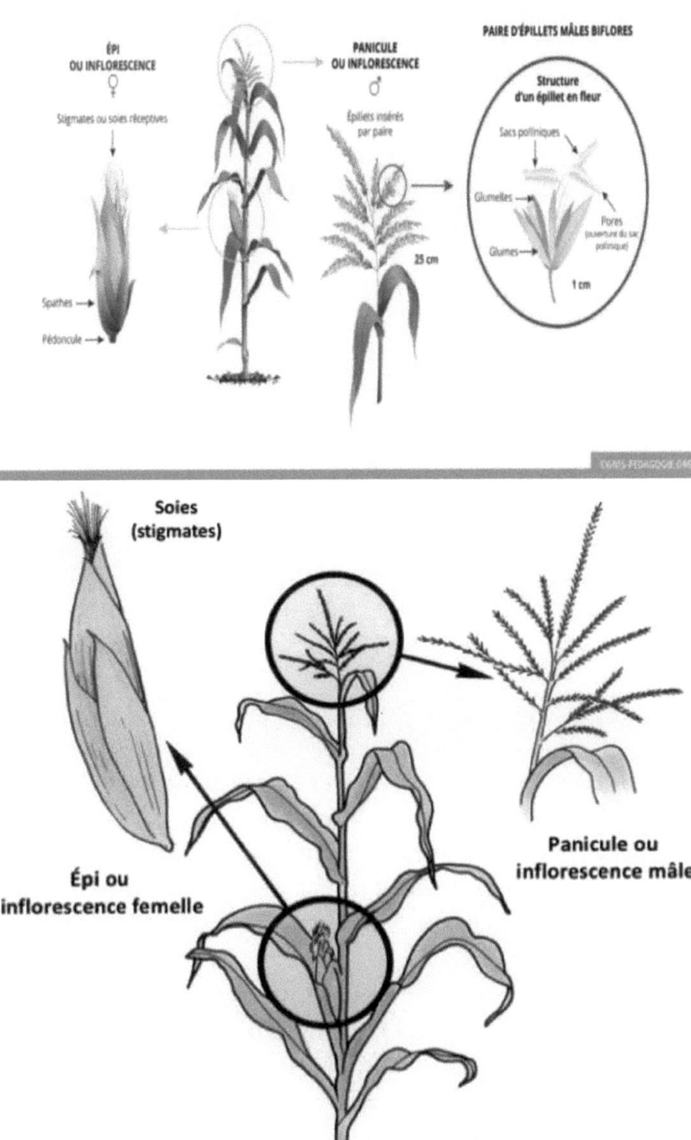

5.5 Fruit

The fruit is the plant organ containing one or more seeds. Characteristic of

Angiosperms, it succeeds the flower by transformation of the pistil. The ovary wall forms the pericarp of the fruit and the ovule gives the seed[94] . It may be a biological fruit or a false fruit (apple, pineapple, etc.). An organic fruit (or false fruit) can be commonly referred to as a vegetable (avocado, tomato, etc.), spice (pepper, chilli pepper, etc.) or cereal (wheat, rice, etc.). The fruit helps the species to reproduce, by protecting the seed or seeds and helping them to spread by animals, in the case of fruit that is generally coloured, sweet (blackberries) or rich in nutrients, by the wind, in the case of fruit with a parachute or wing, or by water, in the case of floating fruit such as coconuts.

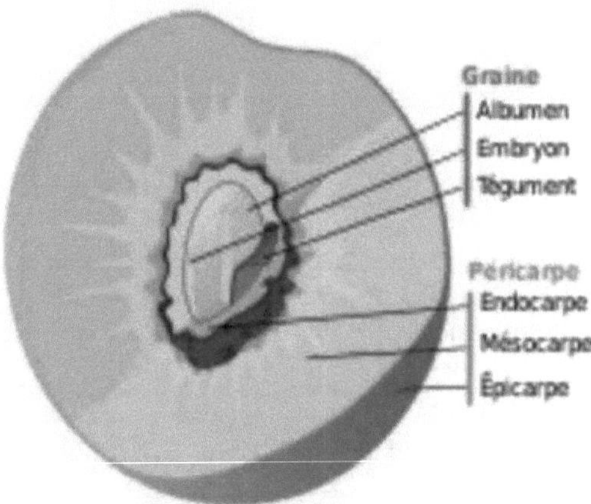

Schematic structure of a typical drupe, the peach, showing both the fruit and the seed.

The fruit produced by the pollinated flower may take the form of a drupe, berry, pod, capsule, achene, etc. The fruit is formed by the transformation of the pistil after fertilisation, or sometimes without fertilisation (this is known as parthenocarpy). More specifically, it is the wall of the ovary (the part of the pistil that contains the ovule) that becomes the wall of the fruit, called the pericarp, surrounding the seeds.

In some cases, the fruit is not the result of the transformation of the pistil and may have a more complex origin, a false fruit. Its formation may result from the transformation of another part of the flower, the floral receptacle. The best-known examples of false fruits are apples and strawberries. It can also result from the transformation of another part of the flower, the carpels, which become drupeoles. These multiple fruits are therefore small agglomerated drupes, known as polydrupes. This is the case with raspberries and blackberries (fruit of the bramble bush). It may result from the transformation of several flowers in an

[94] Bernard Boullard, *Plantes & Champignons*, Éditions Estem, 1997, 878 p.

inflorescence, known as an infrutescence. This is the case, for example, with pineapples, figs and blackberries (fruit of the mulberry tree).

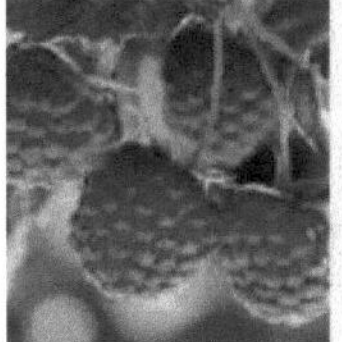
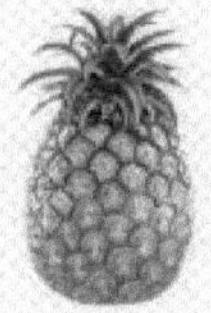
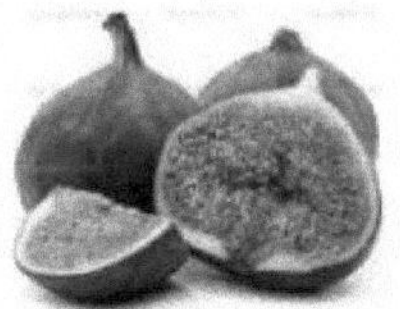
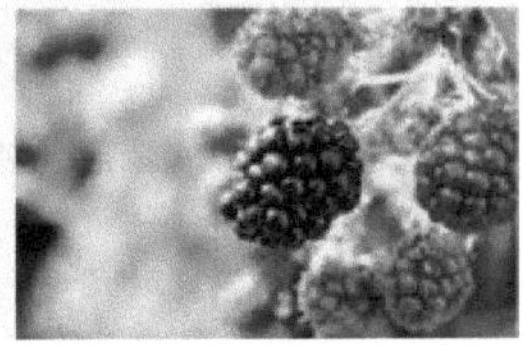

Raspberry Pineapple Fig Blackberry (fruit of the mulberry tree)

The pericarp is made up of three layers: the epicarp, which is generally coloured and usually called the skin; the mesocarp, which gives the juicy part of fleshy fruits; and the endocarp, which is sometimes lignified and called the stone. In botany, the epicarp or exocarp is the outer wall of a fruit. It covers the layer known as the mesocarp. It is generally coloured. It is usually called the skin or peel. In the specific case of citrus fruits, the exocarp is called the flavedo. The mesocarp is the intermediate part of the fruit, commonly known as the *pulp* in the case of fleshy fruits. It is derived from the transformation of the parenchyma of the ovary wall. In the particular case of citrus fruits, the outer part of the mesocarp, which is white and spongy, is called the albedo. The endocarp is the innermost layer of the pericarp, the fruit tissue surrounding the seed. It can be used to distinguish a berry from a dupe among fleshy fruits. If it is sclerified, it forms a stone around the seed (the fruit will be a drupe); if it is not, the seed will be called a pip (the fruit will be a berry). In botany, for example, an avocado is considered to contain a seed and a peach a stone.

In botanical typology, a distinction is made between: fleshy fruits: berries such as grapes, tomatoes, avocados, oranges, etc.; drupe-like fruits such as plums, peaches, olives and cherries. They are characterised by a seed with a hard shell (lignified endocarp). There are also dehiscent dried fruits (which eventually open) such as hellebore and peony. The pod is a characteristic fruit of the Fabaceae, also known as legumes, such as peas, soya, locust trees and alfalfa. A distinction should also be made between fruits with a slit dehiscence capsule (septicide) such as colchicum, tobacco and gentian. There is the loculicidal capsule such as the tulip, lily, violet, silique: Others are paraplacental dehiscence. These are characteristic fruits of brassicas such as cabbage and rape. Others are pyxides, with circular dehiscence, such as chickweed. Some, such as carnations and poppies, have apically dehiscent capsules. Dry, indehiscent fruits (which do not open) are achenes, such as dandelion, valerian and strawberry (a strawberry is a false fruit dotted with brownish achenes). There are also caryopsis fruits, which are characteristic of Poaceae (grasses) such as wheat and maize. Others are samarose, such as maple, ash and elm. Schizocarp fruits contain several achenes: carrot, mint.

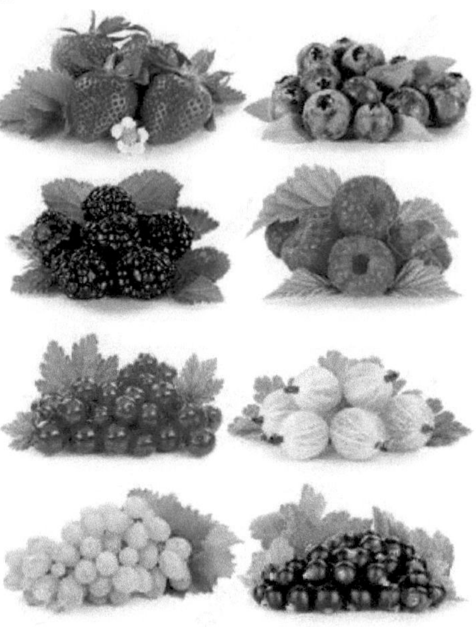

Berries

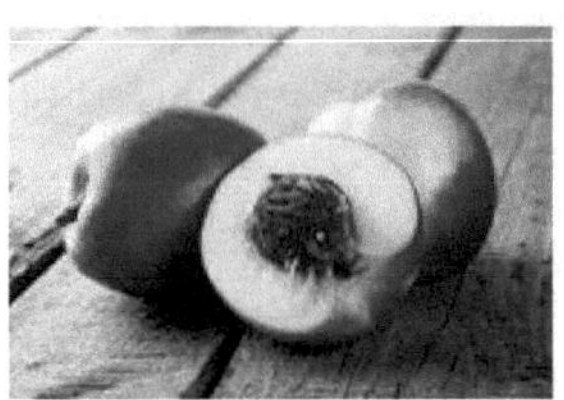

Apple (drupe)

CHAPTER 6

6. Phytomedical and biochemical glossary

We have chosen to provide readers with the meanings of words often encountered in the previous two main sections on plant descriptions, chemical properties, therapeutic properties and dosage. This lexical essay begins with the etymology of the words, followed by their botanical, biochemical and medical usage. In some cases, more detailed explanations will even be given of medicinal plant remedies, in the case of diseases or healing practices. The glossary is presented in alphabetical order.

achene (achene): Latin achena, from Ancient Greek à-, a- (without) and χαινειν khainein (to open, to be gaping, to yawn). In botany, this is the indehiscent fruit, containing only one seed whose pericarp, more or less sclerified, is not fused to the seed. For example: the acorn, the fruit of the oak, is an achene; artichokes and dandelions have feathery achenes. The achene is also the typical fruit of the Fagaceae: beech and chestnut, whose flowers have a multi-locular ovary. In this case, the single seed results from the abortion of unfertilised ovules. Some achenes have outgrowths resulting from the transformation of the style. This is the case with the achene of the Asteraceae, which bears a pappus of hairs used to disperse them in the wind, or the achene of the clematis (buttercups), which bears a long, whitish, feathery style that is very visible in hedges in winter.

*alkaloid***:** Arabic ^[1] ãl-qily (soda), from medieval Latin *alkali, a* plant of the genus Salsola from which a more or less pure sodium carbon was extracted for a long time, known as "soda", from which caustic soda could be made. The term *al qali* was also used, like the French word soude with its dual use for the saliferous plant and the chemical substance soude, to designate calcined ash with basic properties; *alkaloid, al qali* (base or with an alkaline or basic character), Greek suffix - είδης -eidês (kinship, resemblance, form), via the German *alkaloid.* This is the generic name for very many natural substances containing one or more nitrogen atoms in a negative oxidation state, in principle engaged in a ring, and giving them more or less marked basic properties. As bases, they are generally insoluble in water and soluble in apolar organic solvents; as salts, their solubilities are the opposite; they often crystallise in a solid state. The associated biological activities can be intense, with a predilection for the central nervous system (morphine, atropine, ergot alkaloids, etc.). Some are anti-cancer agents (vinblastine, camptothecin, etc.) or anti-parasitic agents (quinine). It is an organic, basic, nitrogenous substance, generally heterocyclic, of plant (rarely animal) origin, endowed with remarkable physiological properties (toxic or therapeutic), such as morphine, nicotine, cocaine, strychnine and quinine. Like a large number of natural products, almost

all common names for alkaloids have an "-ine" ending, such as nicotine, caffeine, atropine, ibogaine, emetine, ergine and morphine. In biological chemistry, alkaloids are usually derivatives of amino acids. They are found in the form of complex mixtures, often based on several or even dozens of different alkaloid molecules, together with their precursors, as secondary metabolites, mainly in plants, fungi and some animal groups. There is one type of alkaloid that contains two nitrogen atoms in the aromatic ring and is not naturally occurring: the pyrazole group. Alkaloids form salts and have a bitter taste. In purified form, the molecules very often reveal an acute toxicity, as well as, in smaller doses, a soothing pharmacological activity, not without habit-forming effects or long-term chronic toxicity. But the minute proportions of caffeine in coffee, cocaine in a dry coca leaf, nicotine in chewing tobacco and nicotine in chewing tobacco have been accepted for their psychotropic, psycoactive, stimulant, doping, tonic, vomiting, calming, sedative and analgesic actions. The best-known pure alkaloid molecules are often highly toxic, as are strychnine, aconitine, atropine and cocaine in measured doses. These include the analgesic properties of morphine or codeine, as part of sedation protocols (anaesthesia) often accompanied by hypnotics, or use as an anti-malarial agent (quinine, chloroquine) or anti-cancer agent (vinblastine, vincristine), and even opiate sedation with ibogaine.
aldehyde: derived from the corresponding hydrocarbon to which the -al ending is added. Methanal, also known as formaldehyde or formaldehyde, is gaseous, but all the other aldehydes are liquid or solid. These compounds are used in industry to manufacture perfumes, medicines, plastics, solvents, paper and textiles. In chemistry, they are organic compounds in which one of the primary carbon atoms carries a carbonyl group. Furfurol (furfural, fural), the raw material for furan resins, is extracted from the bran of certain parts of the corn cob. It is an aldehyde from which furfuryl alcohol (furol) is obtained by hydrogenation. On an industrial scale, the controlled oxidation of primary alcohols can be used to produce aldehydes, taking precautions to ensure that the reaction stops before carboxylic acids are formed. This is how methanal is made from methanol. Aldehydes are also produced on a massive scale from alkenes by hydroformylation, a method often referred to as the oxo process: butanal, for example, is synthesised from propene, carbon monoxide and dihydrogen, in the presence of a catalyst. Because of the strong polarisation of the C=O bond, aldehydes, like ketones, are susceptible to nucleophilic addition on the carbon carrying the function. This property is used to protect the carbonyl function by acetalisation, a reversible process consisting of adding two alcohols to the carbonyl to form an inert compound called an acetal.

alicament: composed of *food* and *medicine*. It is a nutrient intended to treat (or prevent the onset of) certain diseases and incorporated into the normal diet. It is also a food product into which have been introduced elements considered to be particularly beneficial to health. In fact, the term "*alicament*" has its origins in traditional Chinese medicine, which attributes curative virtues to many foods. However, in Western medicine, no food is a substitute for a medicine, although certain foods can help prevent or treat certain illnesses. Alicaments are products of animal or plant origin containing substances that the body needs for nutrition. These substances are proteins, carbohydrates, lipids, water, minerals and vitamins.

There are two types of food used to treat health problems: functional (natural) foods, which are interesting for their natural virtues, and industrial foods, which are foods processed by industrial methods to obtain added beneficial nutritional value.

Natural alicaments are raw, unprocessed foods such as vegetables, fruit and meat. For example: beetroot, which is excellent for the liver, also helps with intestinal transit; celery has antiseptic and rheumatic properties. It protects against cystitis, gout, urinary tract infections, hypertension and arthritis. Parsley protects the kidneys, bladder and prostate. Garlic and onion improve blood circulation and help combat cardiovascular disease. Artichoke stimulates liver cell regeneration. Green tea is an excellent antioxidant. Turmeric has anti-inflammatory and antioxidant properties. Cabbage has anti-inflammatory and diuretic properties, and also helps to lower blood sugar levels. As for processed foods, these are unprocessed products to which nutrients have been added. Examples include: breakfast cereals rich in iron and B vitamins; yoghurts with active bifidus, which are very good for digestion and transit; margarines enriched with Omega 3, which prevent cardiovascular risks. In fact, the potential of health foods is often due to the presence of micronutrients in interesting quantities. These include vitamins C, E, K and B9, pre- and probiotics, dietary fibre and omega-3s.

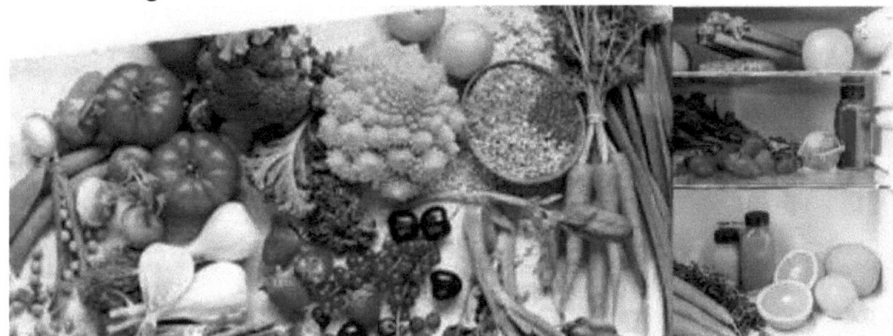

amenorrhoea: from the ancient Greek Ά privative, from μήν, (month), and ρείν, rhein (to flow). It is a condition in which menstruation flows less than usual, or does not flow at all, although there is no pregnancy. This absence of menstruation may be primary or secondary. Primary amenorrhoea is the absence of menstruation at the age of 15 in patients with normal growth and secondary sexual characteristics. Secondary amenorrhoea is the absence of periods for 3 months in the case of regular menstrual cycles, or for at least 6 months in the case of irregular periods. Anatomical causes of amenorrhoea include: congenital anomalies of the female genital tract (e.g. vaginal agenesis, hymen imperforation), acquired anomalies (e.g. Asherman's syndrome or cervical stenosis). Frequent endocrinological causes include: constitutional pubertal delay, pregnancy (most common cause in women of fertile age), polycystic ovary syndrome, hyperprolactinaemia (e.g. due to pituitary adenoma, amenorrhoea due to breastfeeding or antipsychotic medication), functional hypothalamic amenorrhoea (e.g. due to excessive exercise, hypoglycaemia, hypoglycaemia), or a combination of these, due to excessive exercise, eating disorders or stress[95] , hormonal drugs (e.g. oral contraceptives, medroxyprogesterone). Progestin-only contraceptives often cause amenorrhoea. Combined oestroprogestogenic contraceptives can cause amenorrhoea if they are used continuously (without placebo pills or any medication every few weeks) or over a long period (if the endometrium becomes atrophic). Amenorrhoea due to ovulatory dysfunction is usually secondary but can be primary if ovulation never begins, for example due to a genetic disorder. If ovulation never begins, the result is usually delayed puberty and abnormal development of secondary sexual characteristics. Genetic abnormalities that include a Y chromosome increase the risk of ovarian cancer. The most common causes of ovulatory dysfunction are disruption of the hypothalamic-pituitary-ovarian axis. Causes include: hypothalamic dysfunction (in particular functional hypothalamic amenorrhoea); pituitary dysfunction; primary ovarian failure (premature ovarian failure); endocrine disorders that cause an excess of androgens (in particular polycystic ovary syndrome).[96]

---

[95] C M Gordon et als, "Functional hypothalamic amenorrhea: An Endocrine Society Clinical Practice Guideline". J Clin Endocrinol Metab 102 /5 (2017) p. 1413-1439, 2017.

[96] V Joan et al, "Amenorrhea" , The MSD Handbook (MD, University of Virginia Health System; Medical Review Jan. 2023), Accessed

18/06/2023 (https://www.msdmanuals.com/fr/professional/gyn%C3%A9cologie-et-obst%C3%A9trique/ troubles-menstruels/am%C3%A9norrh%C3%A9e):

amylaceous: *From Greek* αμυλον *ámulon* (unmilled), from Latin *amylum* (which gave starch), and the suffix -ase. It refers to an element or organ rich in starch. The starch in plants, for example, is used as an ingredient for the human food and animal nutrition markets, as well as for many non-food industries. These include products such as maize (maizena), rice (rice starch), wheat (wheat starch), manioc (tapioca) and potatoes (potato starch). Semolina is mainly extracted from durum wheat. This ground grain is mainly used to make semolina and little flour. There are also semolinas made from soft wheat, barley, oats, maize and rice. Non-starchy vegetables include artichokes, asparagus, bean sprouts, Brussels sprouts, broccoli, cauliflower, celery, cucumber, aubergine, mushrooms, onions, green salad, spinach, tomatoes, turnips and courgettes. Daddy Starch Icing Sugar is the icing sugar used by pastry chefs, which contains starch to ensure a long-lasting glaze on all pastries.
analgesic: From the Greek αντί, anti (opposed to, against) and άλγος, álgos (suffering) Analgesics are drugs used to eliminate pain such as aspirin, paracetamol and ibuprofen, morphine. Ibuprophen is most effective against certain types of pain, such as toothache and sprains. Its synonym is analgesic.
Anaesthesia: From the Greek prefix άν-, an-, in- (without); from α'ίσθησις, aísthêsis, (sensation, faculty of perceiving through the senses). Anaesthesia is the suppression of sensation (and in particular the sensation of pain). Its purpose is to enable a medical procedure to be carried out that would otherwise be too painful. Anaesthesia can be applied to a limb, a region or the whole body (general anaesthesia). Loco-regional anaesthesia is also used for chronic pain. The field of medicine that studies and practises anaesthesia is anaesthesiology.
anorexia: Ανορεξία, from άν (without, stop, absence of) privative, and ορέγομαι (to desire); from Ancient *Greek* άνορεξία , *anorexía* (appetite). In nutrition, it refers to the lack of appetite or absence of appetite, but it actually means the behaviour that consists of restricting oneself from food. It is a symptom resulting from extremely diverse somatic or psychological causes. In psychiatry, anorexia is one of the main symptoms of the depressive syndrome. In medicine, it is the sensation of satiety that occurs in a number of infectious diseases (cancer, tuberculosis, etc.), digestive tract diseases and other serious illnesses.
anthraquinone: Contraction of *anthracene - a* polycyclic aromatic hydrocarbon with three rings in a row, whose name itself derives from anthracite - and *quinone. In* agricultural and pharmaceutical chemistry, it is the chemical substance derived from anthracene, used as a laxative in medicine and in the

---

1-6.

past as a corvifuge in agriculture. Anthraquinone belongs to the chemical family of polycyclic aromatic hydrocarbons. It is a derivative of anthracene. It occurs naturally in a number of animals and plants, and is also an active substance in plant protection products or pesticides that have a repellent effect on birds. Isolated, it has the appearance of a solid crystalline powder, ranging from yellow and light grey to grey-green. More generally, an anthraquinone is a chemical compound with this motif in its structure. Other names for anthraquinone are 9,10-dihydro-9,10-dioxoanthracene, anthradione, 9,10-anthraquinone and anthracene-9,10-quinone, and its popular names include anthranoid, *hoelite*, *morkit* and *corbit*. Anthraquinone occurs naturally in certain plants such as borage, senna, aloes, rhubarb, a type of North American buckthorn sometimes called cascara, fungi, lichens and most insects, where it serves as the basic skeleton for pigments. Natural derivatives of anthraquinone tend to have laxative effects.

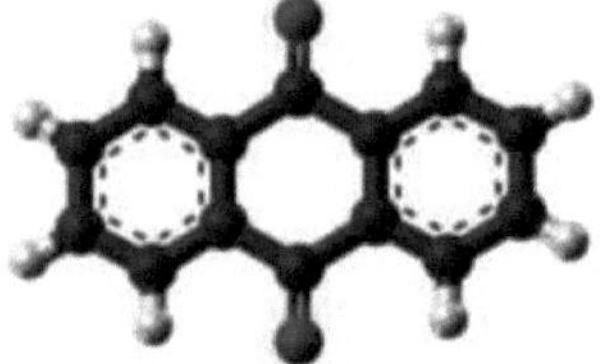

Structure of the anthraquinone molecule.

In medical applications, anthraquinone and its natural derivatives are used to treat functional intestinal disorders such as functional colopathy, laxophobia and constipation. Anthraquinone and its active derivatives, such as anthraquinone glucosides, stimulate peristalsis in the small intestine and increase peristaltic movements in the colon. Anthraquinone glucosides are transformed in the colon into sennosides. Sennosides are hydrophilic and reduce water absorption to ensure a fluid faecal bowl. They therefore prevent the formation of lumpy stools. Anthraquinone is used as a laxative or purgative above a threshold of 30 mg to 36 mg per day. Above this sennoside threshold, stools tend to become very soft or liquid. Anthraquinone sennosides and glucosides contain an aglycone group (glycoside). They are present in the pods and leaves of senna, the rhubarb hhizome, borage, cascara and, in particular, aloes. Prolonged use beyond eight weeks, or abuse, leads to melanism of the colon, due to the release of lipofuscin (present in histiocytes and mast cells) in the colon.

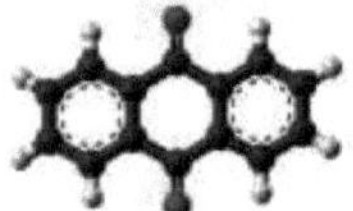

Structure of the anthraquinone molecule

anthelmintic. Vermifuge syrup. Wormwood Artemisia absinthium. Here are a few worm-eating plants: Sea Buckthorn Hippophae rhamnoide; Wormwood Artemisia vulgaris; Aurone Artemisia abrotanum; Nightshade Mirabilis jalapa; Nasturtium Tropaeolum majus; Sea Fennel Crithmum maritimum; Juniper Juniperus oxycedrus. The same applies to garlic and pumpkin seeds. The latter contain an amino acid called cucurbitacin. Other remedies include infusions of dried thyme and spiced decoctions of cinnamon, tinctures of black walnut husk, fresh clove powder and wormwood leaves.

Antibiotic: From the Greek άντί, anti (against, opposed to) and βιος, bios (life, existence). This is the natural or synthetic substance that destroys or blocks the growth of bacteria. In the first case, it is referred to as a bactericidal antibiotic and in the second case as a bacteriostatic antibiotic. When the substance is used externally to kill the bacteria on contact, it is called an antiseptic rather than an antibiotic. The first isolated antibiotics (penicillins) were natural substances produced by a yeast of the genus Penicillium.

anticancerous: From the Greek Άντί (against) and cancer which is from the Sanskrit "karkata", meaning crab, crayfish, or the zodiacal sign of cancer from which the ancient Greek καρκίνος karkinos and then the Latin cancer would derive. All remedies and therapeutic measures used to combat cancer are known as anticancer treatments. The main types of cancer treatment are: surgery, chemotherapy, targeted therapies, radiotherapy, hormone therapy, immunotherapy. All these treatments aim to eliminate cancer cells. They act either locally, i.e. only on the cancer cells in an affected organ, or systemically, i.e. on all the cancer cells present in the body. Targeted therapies are selective and attack a specific target in the cancer cell. Surgery and radiotherapy are local treatments, while chemotherapy and hormone therapy are general treatments. These treatments may be combined to a greater or lesser extent[97] . To combat cancer, the following plants should be consumed: Turmeric, Ginseng, Ginko, Aloe; plants from the Cruciferae family such as Broccoli, radish, Brussels sprouts and other cruciferae containing isothiocyanates (ITCs), which provide defences against the onset of cancer. They act by binding to carcinogenic elements, limiting the development of Helicobacter pilori and reducing chronic inflammation of the stomach, which often generates tumours. A number of epidemiological studies have demonstrated the benefits of turmeric, which destroys cancer cells and, in addition to its anti-oxidant and anti-inflammatory

---

[97] "Cancer: the different types of treatment", consulted on 18/06/2023 (https://www.roche.fr/fr/patients/info-patients-cancer/traitement-cancer/traitements-cancer.html) 13.

action, blocks the formation of new blood vessels that develop to feed tumours and thus cause their death; red ginseng, which in the case of breast cancer limits the spread of cancer cells as a preventive measure or as a complement to anti-cancer treatment; and aloe arborescens, which reduces the number of cancer cells in the liver. It is also thought to prevent this type of cancer thanks to its ability to inhibit the development of cancer cells; gingko bilola reduces cancer cells with its anti-angiogenesis properties and, like turmeric, blocks the formation of new blood vessels, thereby preventing the development of tumours; spirulina, a micro-alga, contains phycocyanin, which delays the development of cancer cells; green tea contains polyphenols: Green tea contains polyphenols, powerful antioxidants and has an anti-inflammatory effect. Above all, it has a preventive effect, particularly against lung cancer[98] .

antidiarrhoeal: Άντί (against), and Διάρροια, from δια (through), and ρείν (to sink). In pharmacology, it is the medicine to combat diarrhoea, relieving its symptoms, but also reducing the risk of dehydration. It may be accompanied by treatment aimed at the cause of the diarrhoea, as in the case of infectious diarrhoea. Patients should drink plenty of water, add plenty of salt to their food and use oral rehydration solutions (ORS). Vegetable products include rice, well-cooked potatoes, pasta and, more generally, anything rich in starch; Roman chamomile, monkey bread pulp and a decoction of the fruit of the African baobab tree (Adansonia digitata).

antihelminthic: Άντί (against) and ελμινς (worm). Sometimes referred to as antihelminthic or vermifuge, it is a class of antiparasitic drugs that combat helminthosis, i.e. destroying helminths (in humans, animals or plants), but it actually more often refers to antiparasitic drugs targeting nematodes and trematodes (Platyhelminthes) likely to parasitise the blood and lymphatic networks, connective tissues or hollow organs (urogenital cavities, lungs. Examples include Syngamus trachea, a haematophagous parasite of bird lungs), as well as all intestinal parasites such as worms (pinworms, roundworms in humans), hookworms, eels and tapeworms.

antipyretic: From ancient Greek πυρετικός , puretikós (of fever, febrile); derived from Άντί, anti- (against) and πυρετός , puretos (fever). Antipyretics or febrifuges are active ingredients used to combat feverish states and certain acute inflammatory syndromes. Their main use is to combat the hyperthermia (rise in body temperature) associated with fever.

---

[98] "Conseils santé. Les plantes qui luttent contre les cancers", MeSoigner.fr, Accessed 18/06 (2023) 1-2 (https://www.mesoigner.fr/conseils/590-les-plantes-qui-luttent-contre-les-cancers).

antirheumatic: From the Greek ἀντί anti (opposite to) and ρευματίζω rheumatizô (to have a cold, rheumatism). It is a substance used to combat rheumatic ailments.
antiscorbutic: From the Greek Ἀντί, anti (against), and medical Latin scorbutus created probably on the basis of Middle Dutch scôrbut, scheurbuik borrowed from Old Swedish skörbjug (Old Norman skyrbjúr composed of skyr (curdled milk, cheese) and bjúr (oedema) which was attributed to the heavy consumption of curdled milk. It is a plant or remedy that combats or prevents scurvy, a disease caused by a lack of vitamin C (ascorbic acid), which in its most serious forms leads to loosening of the teeth and purulent gums, haemorrhaging and, last but not least, scurvy: fumitory, barley malt, potato, blackcurrant berry, menyanthus, sorrel, horseradish, lemon, black mustard, oxalis, rocket, cochlearia, turnip, parsley, rowan, watercress, various oranges, poplar bark and cabbage.
antiseptic: From the Greek Ἀντί, anti- (against, opposed to) from the Latin radical septicus which refers to the Greek σκεπτικός, skeptikós (which putrefies; said of that which produces putrefaction or infection), from σηψις, sépsis (putrefaction). It refers to a product or reagent that destroys bacteria, fungi or viruses, or opposes their multiplication, thus treating or preventing infections or putrefaction. In pharmacology, it is the product used on the external surfaces of the body, which destroys micro-organisms.
antitumoral: From the Greek Ἀντί (against) and the Latin tumor (swelling, puffiness, puffiness), from the verb tumere (to be swollen, swollen). The term antitumour is used to describe all measures and remedies against tumours. A tumour is a lump of varying size caused by an excessive multiplication of normal cells (benign tumour) or abnormal cells (malignant tumour). Benign tumours (e.g. moles, warts) develop locally without affecting neighbouring tissues. Malignant tumours (cancer) tend to invade neighbouring tissues and migrate to other parts of the body, producing metastases. When a tumour is malignant, it invades organs and destroys them. Through the blood and lymphatic vessels, it tries to spread and develop throughout the body, forming secondary tumours known as metastases. This is known as cancer. Here are a few examples of anti-tumour plants: cruciferous plants, red ginseng, aloe arborescens and ginkgo biloba. Vitamin E, which starves breast cancer cells, is the all-time champion. It's found in wheat germ oil, tea, turmeric, lavender, citrus fruits, cabbage (Brassica), red grapes, garlic, soya, berries (especially strawberries), parsley and artichokes. And to kill cancer cells, eat garlic, seaweed, broccoli, coffee, mushrooms, dark chocolate, turmeric, raspberries,

linseed and pomegranate[99] .
apex: is an acronym[100] , originally a Latin word meaning apex or point. The corresponding adjective, apical, describes what is at or near the top or an extremity. In botany, the plant apex is the end of a stem, root, leaf or thallus. Cells divide, elongate and ensure the growth in length of aerial and underground stems: stem apex and root apex respectively. The highest apex is called the "apical zone". The apex is an active zone for gene expression.

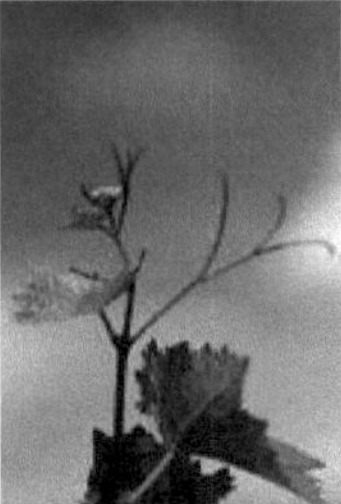

Stem apex with grapevines.

The cauline apex is located at the end of the stem of a plant (apical) or at the nodes on the stem (axial). It is easy to spot because it is here that new leaves are produced. They are the source of auxin, a hormone that inhibits the development of lower buds.

---

[99] O Anne-Sohie, "10 aliments anti-cancer à privilégier", Radis 06/09 (2021) 1-2.

[100] APEX is an acronym. The common noun apex (invariable plural), originally a Latin word (plural apices), means "apex" or "point". The corresponding adjective, apical, describes what is at or near the top or an extremity. In anatomy, it is the tip or apex of a cone-shaped organ. The apex is the botanical term for the end of an organ, in this case the leaf. In other words, it is the apex of the leaf. Acute apex: Leaf where the apex of the blade forms an acute angle. Obtuse apex: Leaf where the apex of the blade forms an obtuse angle.

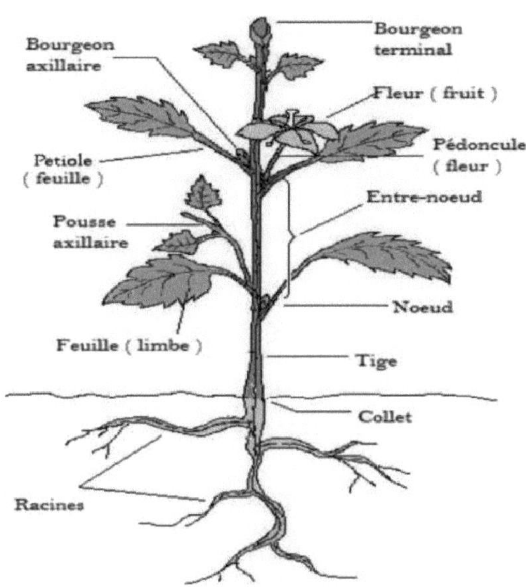

Root apices are located at the end of the main root, or adventitious roots, and are the source of the stimulating hormone cytokinin. A plant apex consists of the following parts (arranged here from the lower part of the root to the upper part): the cap, which protects the apical zone from external aggressions that could be harmful to root growth, but also acts as a guide for the root, by acting as a gravity "sensor", resulting in positive geotropism; it is located at the tip of the root; the quiescent centre, which keeps the meristem cells dividing[101] ; the meristem, which is the zone where new cells are generated to increase the length of the root[102] .

This division of meristem cells involves the process of mitosis, and more generally the cell cycle in a eukaryotic cell; the zone of cell elongation, which corresponds to a zone where cells elongate as a result of various processes (turgor pressure, action of auxin on the cell walls, etc.).

[101] Cell division and elongation in the root apex: diversity of responses to water deficit, PhD thesis, François Bizet, 2014.
[102] Florimond A., Pothet A., "Vegetative meristem" on ens-lyon.fr (accessed 28/06/2023).

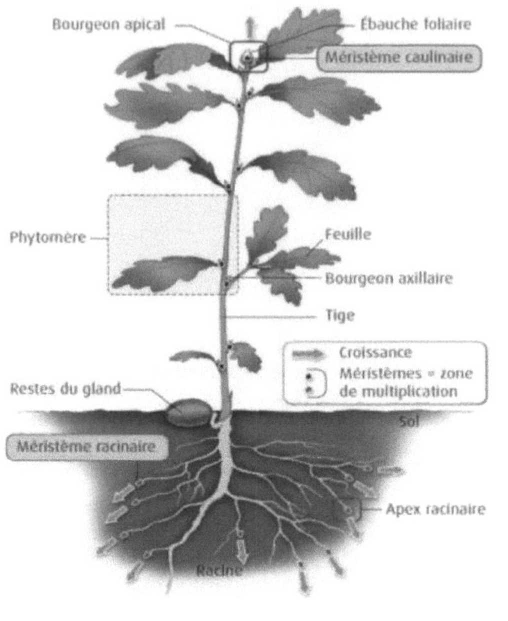

*aphta:*A mouth ulcer is a painful ulceration in the mouth, usually on the inside of the cheeks, which heals spontaneously. It is preceded by a sensation of cooking or burning. This is followed by the appearance of a painful red spot and, very quickly, a rounded or oval ulceration measuring between 2 and 10 mm, with a yellowish or greyish background and a clearly defined red border. Mouth ulcers occur from childhood onwards and are less common after the age of 50. They are favoured by certain foods and fatigue. They do not bleed, but are painful, especially during meals or when brushing your teeth. A canker sore is a single occurrence, but there may be several (up to 6) in a single outbreak. In the mouth, canker sores can occur on all the mucous and mobile areas of the mouth: the edges, underside or tip of the tongue, inside the lips and cheeks, floor of the mouth (under the tongue). The gums attached to the bone, the hard palate and the dry side of the lips are spared from mouth ulcers. Mouth ulcers are not contagious, except in the case of infection. There may be cases of several outbreaks of mouth ulcers per year. This is known as recurrent aphthosis. Canker sores can be miliary when they consist of a large number of canker sores (50 to 100) of very small size, less than one millimetre. Giant canker sores, on the other hand, each measure 1 to 2 cm and can take up to a month to heal. They are different from contagious ulcerative lesions caused by infections: primary herpes infection, chickenpox, hand-foot-and-mouth syndrome, primary HIV infection. Ulcerations of the dental mucosa of the mouth may occur in the event of defective dental care: sharp teeth or dental materials; mucosal wounds associated with the wearing of dento-facial orthopaedic appliances or dental prostheses; dental trauma. Certain factors seem to play a role in the appearance of mouth ulcers: stress and fatigue; certain foods: nuts, peanuts, Gruyère cheese, strawberries, tomatoes, etc.; certain drugs: non-steroidal anti-inflammatory drugs, beta-blockers (heart medication), biphosphonates (drugs used in the treatment of osteoporosis), cancer treatment drugs; the menstrual period for some women.

apoptosis: from ancient Greek ἀπόπτωσις, apóptôsis; from apo, apo (away) and ptosis, (fall). This refers to the phenomenon of natural cell death. It is the process by which cells trigger their self-destruction in response to a signal. It is one of the possible pathways of physiological cell death, genetically programmed and necessary for the development and survival of multicellular organisms. Its balance with cell proliferation allows tissue homeostasis. Unlike necrosis, it does not cause inflammation: the plasma membranes are not destroyed, at least initially, and the cell emits signals (in particular, it exposes phosphatidylserine, a phospholipid normally found in its inner leaflet, on the outer leaflet of its plasma membrane) which allow it to be phagocytosed by white blood cells, particularly macrophages.

apyrexia: απυρεξια, from gre α- privative (without), from ancient Greek πυρεσσειν, puressein (to have a fever), from ancient Greek πυρ (fire, fever). It is the absence of fever or the absence of a rise in normal body temperature (around 37°C). When we list a patient's symptoms, we say, depending on the case, that they are febrile or apyretic. When a patient's fever falls, they become apyretic. An antipyretic drug is a product which, like paracetamol, fights fever, in other words achieves apyrexia.

Asthma: from the Greek ἅσθμα, ásthma, via the Latin asthma (difficult breathing). It is a disease of the respiratory system affecting the lower airways and in particular the bronchioles, defined as breathing discomfort on exhalation. It is a respiratory condition characterised essentially by difficult breathing accompanied by a wheezing noise and by bouts of intense suffocation.

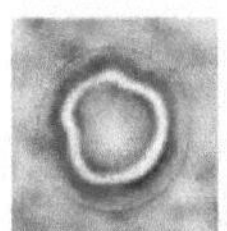
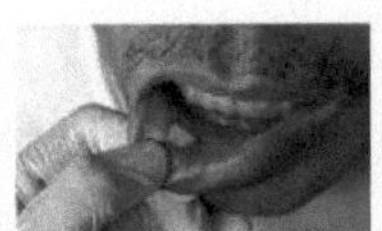
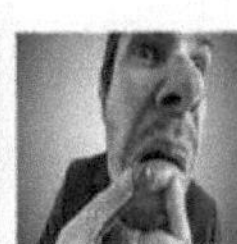
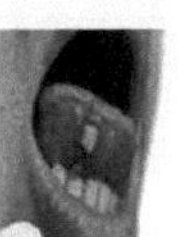
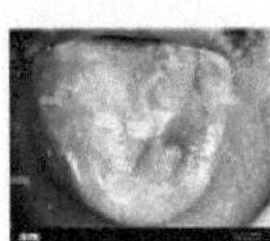

Berry: A berry is a fleshy fruit containing one or more seeds called pips, but it cannot be opened: the berry is therefore said to be indehiscent. Berries include blackcurrants, redcurrants, grapes, bilberries, cranberries, raspberries, black cherries, white mulberries, blackberries, wild strawberries, cranberries, gooseberries, tomatoes and kiwi fruit. If the ovary wall is thin and has little moisture around the seed, the fruit is dry. If, on the other hand, the ovary wall is succulent (full of water, sugars, pigments and other substances), the fruit is said to be "fleshy": berry or drupe.

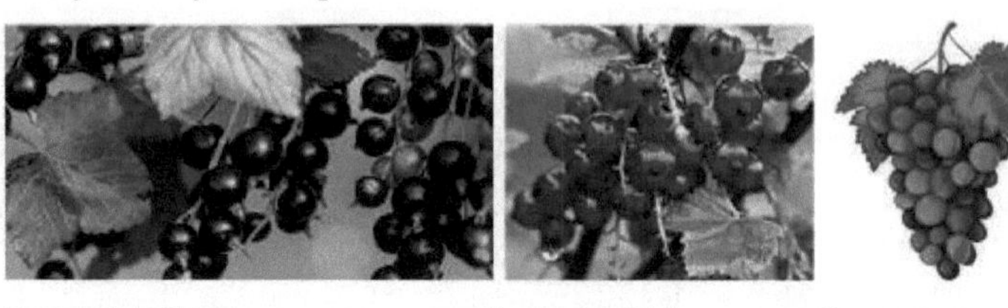

Baie de cassis ***de groseille*** ***de raisin***

Blackcurrant currant grape berry

brède: From Latin blitum, ancient Greek βλίτον, blíton, through Portuguese bredo (leaf, herb in regional French (as in Madagascar). In botany, it is a leaf that is edible after cooking and is used in East Africa in stews. Brèdes are also herbs or green vegetables cooked al dente, often with garlic, ginger and onions. They are a variety of leafy vegetables mainly cooked in the Mascarene Islands, Seychelles and Madagascar.
calciferol: From the Greek χάλιξ, khálix, genitive χάλικος, khálikos, small stone, pebble, limestone, lime, Latin calx, genitive calcis, small stone, pebble used for playing, lime, Latin ferre to bear, to support, to present, to carry, to report, to tell, to hawk, to obtain, to carry away, to produce, to set in motion, to direct, to lead, suffix - ol alcohol function. This is vitamin D, which helps to fix calcium. Insufficient levels cause rickets (a bone growth disease), while excessive levels cause diarrhoea and excessive ossification. There are two molecules accepted as nutritional vitamin D: vitamin D2 (ergocalciferol) and vitamin D3 (cholecalciferol).
cancer: This word comes from the Sanskrit karkata, meaning crab, crayfish, or the zodiacal sign of cancer from which the ancient Greek καρκίνος, karkinos and then the Latin cancer would derive. Cancer is a disease caused by the transformation of cells that become abnormal and proliferate excessively. These dysregulated cells eventually form a mass that is called a malignant tumour. Cancer cells tend to invade neighbouring tissues and detach from the tumour. They then migrate via blood vessels and lymphatic vessels to form another tumour (metastasis).
carminative: From the Latin carminare (to card wool), transformed in medieval

Latin into carminativus (to disperse by scraping), hence to purify, to cleanse by eliminating. A carminative food is one that encourages the expulsion of intestinal gases, while reducing their production. Carminative plants include ginger, garlic, peppermint, fennel, fragrant dill, green anise, basil, cardamom, chervil, coriander, tarragon, hyssop, marjoram, nutmeg, onion, savory, sage, thyme, wild angelica and star anise. Herbal medicine combines choleretic and cholagogic plants (respectively: which promote the production of bile by the liver; which promote the excretion of bile) with carminative plants to relieve digestive disorders, particularly constipation.

cataplasm: from Latin cataplasma, from Greek κατάπλασμα, from κατά, (on, against, according to) and πλάσμα, (application), from πλάσσειν (apply, form). In herbalism, a poultice is a plant preparation that is pasty enough to be applied to the skin for therapeutic purposes. The plant can be ground, chopped hot or cold or mixed with linseed meal to obtain the right consistency. The classic flaxseed meal poultice is prepared using water mixed with cold flaxseed meal. Cook gently, stirring constantly to obtain the desired consistency. A green clay poultice can also be made from powder diluted in water and applied in a layer to the area to be treated before wrapping with a damp cloth or bandage. The poultice should act as a support for the substances that will be deposited on the surface when it is applied.

cauterize: From Latin cauterizare, derived from Ancient Greek καυτηριάζω, kautêriázô (to mark with a red-hot iron). This is a surgical term that involves the application of a fire-reddened iron, to parts of the body. The instruments used are known today as cauteres. The use of the current cauteres is to consume the decay of the bones, to prevent the vermoulure which this disease can cause while progressing. Their application, by drying up the moisture or sanitis that exudes from decayed bones, causes exfoliation and leads to solid healing of the ulcer, with a good scar. Current cauteres are applied by reddening their front end in a blazing fire. Deep decay requires a stronger application of cauteres than superficial decay, because to obtain the expected results, it is necessary to burn all the healthy parts, in order to dry out and dry up the vessels from which the gnawing serosities come.

cirrhosis: From the ancient Greek κιρρός, kirrhós (red) due to the granular, reddish-yellow production caused by the disease, and the suffix -ose. Cirrhosis is a serious liver disease that irreversibly damages this digestive organ. Alcohol consumption is the main cause. It can also occur as a result of chronic viral hepatitis, hepatic steatosis (non-alcoholic fatty liver) or a rare disease.

Corns: These are small, thickened areas of skin on the feet, in two parts: a rounded, horny, dense and translucent core, visible under the skin of the foot; a tip in the shape of an inverted cone, which penetrates the deep layers of skin opposite the bony protrusion under the horn. The hard horn is a type of horn that has the particularity of being rigid. It is rather yellowish in colour, transparent and more or less massive, often giving the impression of a pebble in the shoe. It can be lodged under the foot, the heel, on the front of the foot, between the toes, in the nail grooves or even under the nails. A hard callus can bleed, inflame or become infected. Soft corns are flexible. It is generally found in areas where there is a lot of maceration, for example between the toes. It can vary in colour, but generally takes on a whitish tinge. It is commonly known as a partridge's eye between the toes. Soft corns can bleed, become inflamed or even become infected.

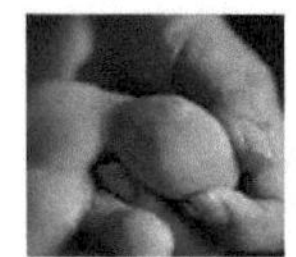
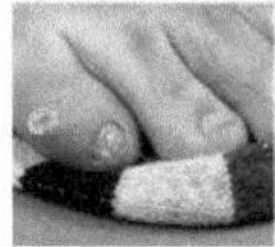
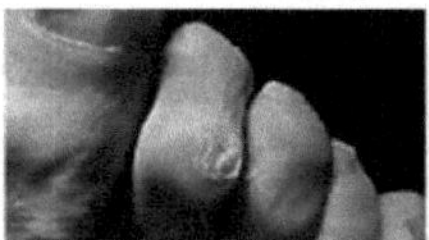
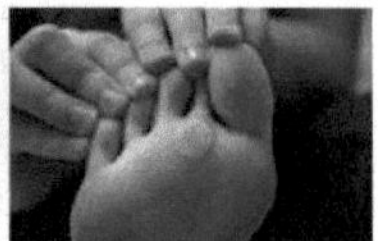

oeil de perdrix

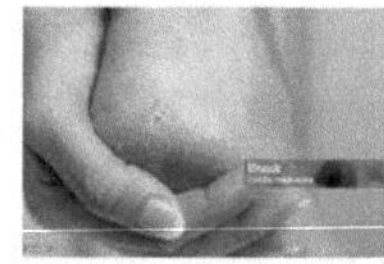
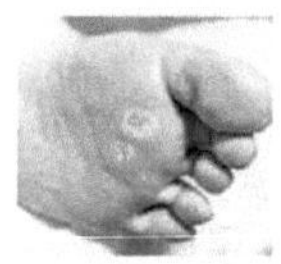

durillon ***Cors***

partridge eye
callus

The difference between corns, calluses and partridge eyes is the location of the hyperkeratosis on the foot. Between the toes, it is called a *partridge eye*. On the tops of the toes, it is called *corns*. Under the sole of the foot, a *callus*.

decoction: from the Latin decoctionem, from coquere (to cook). This is the process of boiling a medicinal substance, usually a plant, in a liquid in order to extract its active principle. It is also a medicinal composition obtained by boiling plant or animal substances in water or another liquid. Example: decoction of plants, roots; decoction of couch grass, cinchona; aperitif decoction, white, emollient[103] ; decoction of
Abrus[104] pecatorius, Cajanus Cajan[105] , Canavalia basiliensis, Crotalaria retusa[106]

[103] Pierre Grenand et al. Papilionaceae à Rutaceae " Pharmacopées Traditionnelles en Guyanne, (Marseilles 2004) p. 520-609.

[104] Creole name: ti panacoco.

[105] Creole names: pois d'angole, pois d'Angola, pois en gaules, West Indian

, Dalbelgia monetaria[107] , Dalbergia riedelit, Desmodium axillare[108] , Dioclea guanensis, Dioclea virgata, Dipteryx odorata[109] , Dipteryx punctata[110] .

Diptera: From Latin *dipteros*, borrowed from Ancient Greek δίπτερος, dipteros (having two wings) by extension "with two rows of columns", composed of δι- , from δίς (dis) "twice" and πτερόν, pteron (wing). It is an order in the class of insects. It is one of the dominant orders in terms of number of species. There are more than 150,000 species of flies. This group includes species known by the vernacular names of flies, hoverflies, mosquitoes, horseflies, midges, etc.

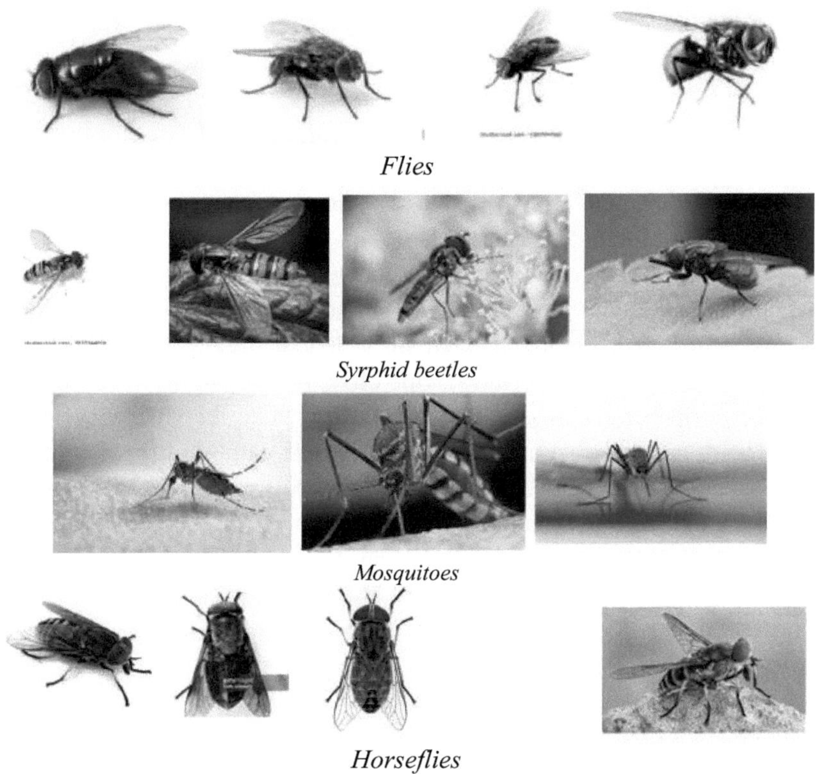

Flies

Syrphid beetles

Mosquitoes

Horseflies

Creole: pois congo.

[106] Creole names: graine chacha [grenn-chacha] (Guyanese), tchak tchak [grenn-tjaktjak] (sainte- lucien), sonnette (West Indian).

[107] Creole names: soumaké, véronique.

[108] Creole name: radié cousin.

[109] French names: faux gaïac (tree, but mainly wood), fève tonka (fruit).

[110] French name: fève tonka.

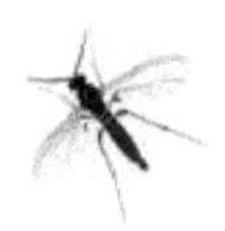 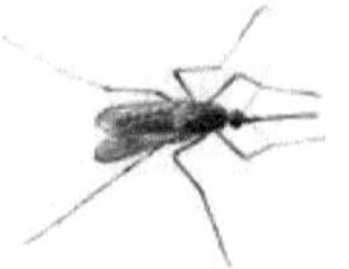 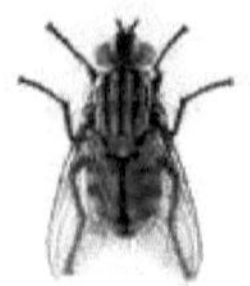 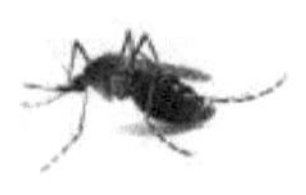

Gnats

Around fifty of these families are important because of their role in the transmission of parasites or pathogens to humans or livestock (Culicidae),

Simulidae, Glossinidae, Phlebotominae, Ceratopogonidae, Huttonidae) of myases (Calliphoridae...) or as crop pests (Cecidomyiidae, Agromyziadae (leafminers), Tephritidae (fruit flies), Psilidae...) or on the contrary as crop beneficials (Syrphidae in part, Tachinidae...).

diuretic: From Low Latin diureticus, itself from Ancient Greek διουρητικός, from δια, dia (through) and οὐρείν, ouréin (to piss). Said of a medicine, remedy, food, action, drink, plant, powder, herbal tea that promotes or stimulates urinary excretion. Examples: redcurrant leaves taken as tea; grape juice that has not yet fermented; new wine that warms up; sweet white wine. Other plants include: dandelion (Taraxacum officinale), hawthorn, horsetail, juniper, parsley, hibiscus, orthosiphon, birch, birch, red pincushion, nettle[111] .

drupe: from the Latin drupa (oliva), ripe olive, itself from the Greek δρύππα / drúppa, overripe olive). It is a fleshy stone fruit, like the cherry, apricot and olive. The drupe arises from a pistil with a single carpel, of the non-adherent "infere" type. In the case of flowers with several free carpels, the result is a multiple, or polydrupe, such as the blackberry or raspberry. The drupe is generally indehiscent (dehiscence not being necessary in the case of a fleshy fruit whose flesh rapidly decomposes, releasing the stone). The drupe is characterised by a pericarp made up of a fleshy part (the mesocarp, called the sarcocarp, covered by the membranous epicarp), which is succulent or fibrous (e.g. the coconut mesocarp), and a sclerotized, i.e. hard, part (the endocarp, called the sclerocarp, which forms the stone). Some fruits, made up of multiple small drupes or "drupelets" agglomerated together, are polydrupes. This is the case with raspberries and blackberries. In the case of fruits of the Rubus genus (raspberries, brambleberries), the fruit arises from a single flower whose pistil is formed from multiple free carpels. Mulberries, on the other hand, which are very similar to brambleberries, are produced from compact catkin-like inflorescences, each drupeole being produced from a different flower.

---

[111] Marie-Céline Ray, "10 plantes diurétiques", La Nutrition. Bon à manger, bon à savoir 19/11 (2020) 1-2.

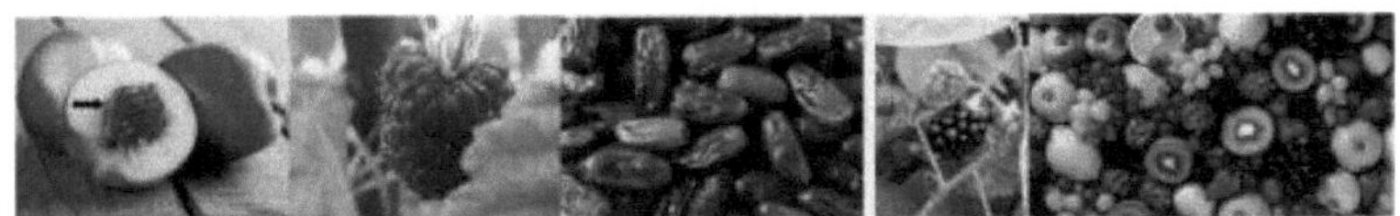

Apple/raspberry/date drupe Blackberry polydrupe/ Fruit polydrupe

dysmenorrhoea: From the ancient Greek δυσ-, dus- (which expresses an idea of difficulty, bad condition), μήν, mèn (month) and ρέω, rheo (to flow). Algomenorrhoea (from the Greek ἄλγος, algos pain) is sometimes referred to as painful menstruation. It refers to the difficulty of menstrual flow. These pains precede or accompany menstruation and may be accompanied by diarrhoea, vomiting, dizziness and headaches.

dyspepsia: From the Latin dyspepsia, borrowed from the ancient Greek δυσπεψία , dyspepsia (indigestion), composed of the prefix δυσ-, dys- and πέψη, pepsè (digestion). Dyspepsia corresponds to a set of symptoms of pain or discomfort in the epigastric area (upper abdomen) originating in the stomach or nearby structures.

Emmenagogue: From the ancient Greek ἔμμηνα, emmena (menstrual); derived from μήν, mèn (month) and ἀγογός agogos (driver). Medicinal plants that stimulate blood flow in the pelvic region and uterus and can treat dysmenorrhoea or amenorrhoea are called emmenagogues. Plants such as yarrow (Achillea millefolium), wormwood (Artemisia absinthium), mugwort (Artemisia vulgaris), parsley (Petroselinum crispum), angelica (Angelica archangelica), nutmeg (Myristica fragrans) and ginger (Zingiber) are used by women to stimulate the onset of menstruation.

enteritis: From the Greek εντερον, enteron (intestine) and -ῖτις , -îtis (inflammation). It is the inflammation of the mucous membrane of the small intestine. It can be acute, chronic, choleriform, infectious, tubercular.

Epilepsy: Greek ἐπιληψία, epilepsia from ἐπί, epi (on), and λαμβάνειν, Iambanein (to take). This is the disorder of the nervous system characterised by repeated seizures involving the sudden onset of convulsions or resulting in various sudden and transient manifestations. It is generalised, when a loss of consciousness is added to convulsions affecting all the muscles of the body. It is partial or focal, when only a group of muscles is involved, at least at the start of the seizure. Temporal epilepsy is that which is accompanied by various disorders of language, vision or hearing. Haut mal" or "grand mal" is a classic form of generalised epilepsy. Petit mal" refers to minor forms of epilepsy, characterised, for example, by a brief loss of consciousness.

febrifuge: From the Latin febris (fever) with the suffix -fuge, from the verb fugare, (makes flee). This refers to any medicine used directly to stop fever, or to destroy its cause and effects. It is not an illness in itself, but a symptom or clinical manifestation of an underlying infection or illness. To recognise symptoms without a thermometer, here are some signs: shivering or sweating, high temperature, rapid pulse, loss of appetite, muscle pains or aches, tiredness, general malaise and headaches, confusion, discomfort with light and certain smells, lack of appetite. A mild fever, or febrile state, occurs when the body temperature is between 37.8°C and 37.9°C[112] . When the temperature is extremely high, over 41.5°C, the condition is called hyperpyrexia. Here are a few febrifuge plants: white willow, meadowsweet, small knapweed and black elder, water hemp (Lycopus Europaeus), thatch (Centaurea calcitrapa), chlorette (Blackstonia perfoliata), gentian (Gentianella campestris), yellow germander (Teucrim flavium), smooth germander (Teucrim lucidum)[113] .

fever (pyrexia): From the Latin febris (fever). Fever is caused by pyrogenic substances released by cells or germs during states of inflammation. Fever is thought to be a defence system designed to inhibit bacterial growth. Pyrogens act on the thermoregulation centre, shifting the thermal equilibrium point upwards: the body is perceived as too cold, which activates thermogenesis (muscle shivering, vasoconstriction). When the fever falls, the set point returns to normal and the body is too hot, triggering thermolysis (vasodilation, sweating). Fever is very often the result of a viral infection, which is generally benign (strep throat, nasopharyngitis, childhood illnesses, bronchitis). Other infectious causes include: bacterial infections, which can affect all organs: nervous system, mouth and respiratory tract, digestive tract, urinary tract, skin, etc. Parasitic infections (malaria when returning from a trip), fungal infections (mushrooms) in immunocompromised people. Non-infectious causes include: vascular causes such as thrombo-embolic venous disease (phlebitis, pulmonary embolism) and heart attacks; certain inflammatory diseases: lupus erythematosus, rheumatoid arthritis, chronic inflammatory bowel disease; cancer, hyperthyroidism, certain allergic reactions and vaccinations.

friction: From the Latin frictio (the action of rubbing). This involves rapid, energetic and repeated rubbing of a part of the body, dry or otherwise, with the hands, a brush or a paddle, for therapeutic purposes (to facilitate the absorption of a medicine by the skin or to increase circulation locally, to soothe a pain, etc.).

flavonoid: From flavedo, derived from the Latin flavus, (yellow) and the Greek

---

[112] Sarah Adida, "Fever: what is it? When to worry", Passeport Santé 28/12 (2022) 1-2.

[113] "Plants with properties: febrifuge", Génial Végétal, consulted on 26/06/2023. (https://www.genialvegetal.net/+-Plantes-propriete-febrifuge-+) p. 1-3.

είδης-eidês suffix (marking kinship, resemblance, appearance)[114] , used in medicine to describe icterus and the yellow appearance in general[115] before designating the outer layer of orange peel[116] or lemon peel[117] . Flavonoids (or bioflavonoids) are secondary metabolites of vascular plants, all sharing the same basic structure formed by two aromatic rings linked by three carbons: C6-C3-C6, a chain often closed to form a hexagonal or pentagonal oxygenated heterocycle. They are real food sources with flavones: naringin, naringenin, hesperetin, eriodictyol, epigallocatechin gallate are found mainly in cabbage, bananas, kiwi fruit, garlic, olives, onions, sprouted seeds and lemons; with flavonols: epigallocatechin, epicatechin, catechin, luleotin in green tea, red wine, grapes, cocoa beans, apricots, berries, apples; with flavones : nobiletin, diosmin, apigenin, wogonin in kiwi, green tea, oregano, spinach, lettuce, broccoli, watermelon, peas, camomile flower, orange, grapes, pumpkin, chickpeas, brown rice, rosemary. For nobelitine, see shikuwasa; with flavonols: Morine, galangin, kaempferol, malvidin in peas, grape seeds, apples, citrus fruit, soya, onions, cucumber, strawberries, tomatoes; with anthocyanins: Cyanidin, hirsutidin, pelargonidin, genistein in red, purple and blue berries, red grapes, pomegranates, red apples, apricots, black beans, red cabbage, purple carrots, aubergines, coloured potatoes, red onions, red or purple radishes, coloured cereals; with isoflavones: Glycitein, equol, daidzein, in soya, soya-based preparations, legumes, parsley, tofu, broad beans, red clover.

In particular, they are pigments involved in the colouring of petals and pericarps, giving a range of colours from ivory to cream (flavones and flavonols), from yellow to orange (chalcones and aurones) and from red to blue (anthocyanins). These are also internal and external photoprotection molecules[118] and have other roles. As soon as they "emerged from the water", plants abandoned the metabolic pathway of mycosporine analogue amino acids and developed a phenolic metabolism, more specifically that of flavonoids, which is an important part of the plant strategy for combating biotic and abiotic

[114] K. Ghedira, "Flavonoids: structure, biological properties, prophylactic role and therapeutic uses", Phytotherapie, vol. 3 4 (2005) p. 162, (DOI 10.1007⁄s10298-005-0096-8).

[115] Œuvres complètes de Philippe Aureolus Theophraste Bombast de Hohenheim, dit Paracelse, vol. 2, Bibliothèque Chacornac,(1914) p. 192.

[116] K. Ghedira, "Flavonoids: structure, biological properties, prophylactic role and therapeutic uses", Phytotherapie, vol. 3 4 (2005) p. 162 (DOI 10.1007/s10298-005-0096-8).

[117] Carl von Linné, Hortus Upsaliensis, exhibens plantas exoticas, Laurentii Salvii (1748) p. 236

[118]D. H. Barker et als, "Internal and external photoprotection in developing leaves of the CAM plant Cotyledon orbiculata", Plant, Cell & Environnement, vol. 20 5 (1997) pp. 617-624 (DOI 10.1111/j.1365- 3040.1997.00078.x).

stresses (exposure to UV rays or cold, wounds, nutrient deficiencies, defending palnts against herbivores and pathogens, etc.)[119] . Flavonoids are naturally present in many plants such as passionflower, aubergine, meadowsweet, St John's wort, blackcurrant, ginkgo biloba, tea, cocoa, red vine, witch hazel, horse chestnut, horsetail and St John's wort.

In therapeutic applications, flavonoids have the ability to neutralise the free radicals that cause oxidative stress, damaging our cells and accelerating ageing. Added to this are their antioxidant effects, which help our bodies to combat potentially dangerous molecules. The benefits of flavonoids, also known as *vitamin P*, include anti-inflammatory, immunostimulant and antioxidant effects. They considerably strengthen all blood vessels, improving circulation. Pycnogenol, derived from Landes pine bark, protects the vascular wall, strengthening it and preserving its resistance. By strengthening the vascular wall, the serous liquid in the blood does not 'leak' through the vascular wall, preventing swelling due to accumulation. When there is a lack of flavonoids, the vascular wall eventually degrades until it ruptures, and varicose veins eventually appear. In women, taking flavonoids such as pycnogenol and rutin can correct leg problems that may be caused by female hormones or the use of the contraceptive pill, with hormonal influences passing from mother to daughter and appearing during typically female events such as pregnancy and the menopause. Flavonoids They have qualities that help regulate life. They are present in the diets of certain traditional cultures.

The function of flavonoids in plants is to give them an attractive colour. They are responsible for the varied colour of flowers and fruit. In leaves, these components are increasingly recognised as stimulating the plant's physiological survival capacity by protecting it against fungal diseases and ultra-violet rays. They are produced during photosynthesis, and their primary role is to protect the leaves from the sun's harmful rays. Before the leaves fall, these bodies are transported by the descending sap and stored in the trunk and roots (e.g. pycnogenol). This colour is even more pronounced in the roots, which are also particularly rich in flavonoids. In spring, before the buds burst, the newly flavonoid-laden sap envelops the buds, protecting them from harmful rays on the one hand and bacteria and viruses that could attack them on the other. As soon as they are born and during their growth, the young shoots are enveloped in sap, and this is when the bees will harvest them. The young leaves in turn produce flavonoids during photosynthesis, and the process continues.

---

[119] DH Barker et als, "Internal and external photoprotection in developing leaves of the CAM plant Cotyledon orbiculata", p. 617-624

Basic propolis, the kind found in a normal beehive, contains around ten flavonoids. While this is enough for bees, it is not enough for humans. No fewer than 25 different flavonoids are needed to maintain a person's health. The main qualities of flavonoids are: antibacterial, antiseptic antiviral and antioxidant,
immunostimulant, anti-allergic, anti-cancerous, antihistaminic, anti-thrombotic and vascular tonic. You can find quercetin, rutin, pycnogenol, grape seed extract and propolis pulver C Lund Aagaard in the shops.
fungal: From the Latin *fungus* (fungus) with the suffix -ique. A fungal infection is caused by parasitic fungi. Candidiasis, caused by the fungus Candida, is the most common vaginal infection. Fungal skin infections can cause redness, itching, scaling and swelling. Other symptoms include coughing, fever, chest discomfort and muscle pain. These infections generally occur after inhalation of fungal spores, which can cause pneumonia as the first sign of infection. As fungal spores are often present in the air or on the ground, fungal infections often begin in the lungs or on the skin. They are rarely serious and progress slowly. Fungi can develop in two forms: yeasts: individual round cells, moulds: several cells forming long narrow filaments called hyphae. They reproduce by spreading microscopic spores that are often present in the air and soil, and can be inhaled or deposited on the surface of the entire body, mainly the skin. Localised fungal infections affect only one area of the body, usually the skin, and the eyes, vagina or mouth. Systemic fungal infections can affect organs such as the lungs, eyes, liver, brain and skin. Opportunistic fungal infections take advantage of a weakened immune system. For this reason, they usually occur in people with weakened immune systems, such as those with AIDS, or those taking drugs that suppress the immune system. Opportunistic fungal infections are found all over the world: aspergillosis, candidiasis, mycormyosis[120] .
friction: From the Latin frictio (the action of rubbing). This involves rapid, energetic and repeated rubbing of a part of the body, dry or otherwise, with the hands, a brush or a paddle, for therapeutic purposes (to facilitate the absorption of a medicine by the skin or to increase circulation locally, to soothe a pain, etc.).
glycaemia: From the ancient Greek γλυκύς, glukús (soft, sweet) and αίμα , haima (blood). This is the sugar content of the blood, which sugar is essentially represented by glucose. In a normal, fasting adult, blood glucose is between 0.80 and 1 g/l. Glucose comes from the various bones provided by food, from glycogen reserves in certain tissues (liver, muscle) (by glycogenolysis) and from

Sonjay G. Revankar, "Presentation of fungal infections", *The MERCK Manual* 04 (2021) p. 1-3.

non-carbohydrate organic nutrients or their derivatives (by gluconeogenesis). It is used by the body either to cover its energy needs or to be stored in the form of muscle or liver glycogen (glycogeno-formation) and lipids.
Carbohydrate: From the ancient *Greek γλυκύς, glukús* (sweet) and *eidos* (form, appearance): In biochemistry and nutrition, this is the type of molecule made up of carbon, hydrogen and oxygen, one of the essential constituents of living beings which corresponds to the sugar molecules.

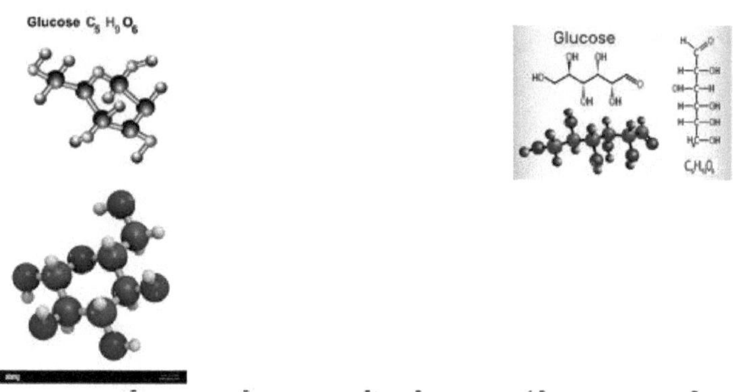

Chemical structure of glucose sugar (dextose, D- glucose) glucose (beta-D-glucose, grape sugar)

Carbohydrates, or slow and fast sugars, are the body's preferred suppliers of energy. In other words, they are the nutrients from which the body draws its energy in a preferential and rapid manner. A distinction is made between :
-*monosaccharides*: glucose, fructose (fruit sugar) and galactose (milk sugar)
-*disaccharides*: sucrose (industrial sugar, made up of glucose and fructose), lactose (carbohydrate found in mammalian milk)
-*oligosaccharides*: raffinose (composed of one galactose unit, one glucose unit and one fructose unit)
-*polysaccharides,* also known as complex carbohydrates: amylopectin (plant starch), glycogen (animal starch), inulin (produced by many types of plant). Polysaccharides are in fact fructose-type sugars linked together. The first three groups of carbohydrates belong to the *simple carbohydrate* family, while the last group belongs to the *complex carbohydrate* family.
Their main source is plants, in dried fruit, fresh fruit, cereals, wholemeal bread, honey, wholemeal sugar and tubers. Carbohydrates are also present in milk and eggs. Egg yolks contain fats, proteins, carbohydrates, minerals, vitamins and water. Water makes up 48% of the total mass of the yolk.

GLUCIDES
10 GRAMMES
=
Miel/Confiture
15 g
Yaourt nature
Yaourt au fruits
200 g 70 g
Pain blanc
20 g
Pain complet
25 g
Pommes de terre
70 g
Riz cuit
45 g
Pâtes cuites
40 g
Pommes chips
20 g
Kit Kat/Mars
15 g
Dattes séchées
13 g
Orange
90 g
Raisin
60 g
Fraise
120 g
Pomme/Poire
70 g
Banane
45 g

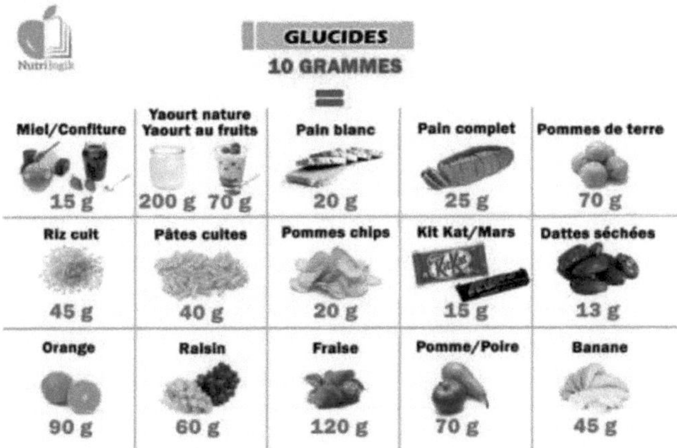

It should be noted, however, that sugar in the strict sense of the term belongs to the carbohydrate family, but not all carbohydrates are strictly speaking sugars. It's a question of belonging, not equivalence. And *sugars* do not necessarily refer to everything that tastes sweet, but simply to carbohydrates, which are a combination of sugar molecules that do not necessarily taste sweet as we know it. Simple carbohydrates, also known as 'sugars' on consumer product labels, are small molecules (low molecular weight) that taste sweet. They include glucose, fructose, lactose, maltose, galactose and sucrose. Simple carbohydrates from fruit are in relatively small quantities and are different from simple carbohydrates from industrial products.

Complex carbohydrates are very large molecules (high molecular weight) with no sweet taste. They include :

-maltodextrins: a combination of several carbohydrates produced by the hydrolysis of wheat or maize starch.

- fructo-oligosaccharides: composed of two simple sugars, glucose and fructose.
- Starch: a mixture of two polysaccharides, amylose and amylopectin. Polysaccharides are complex carbohydrates made up of a large number of simple sugars linked together by glycosidic bonds.
- Cellulose: a polysaccharide made up of numerous glucose molecules, which is a fibre that forms part of the structure of plants.
- Pectins: an acidic polysaccharide found in plants and used as a gelling agent.
- and fibre: starchy polysaccharides that are not broken down by digestive enzymes. Fibre is therefore also a complex carbohydrate, except that it is not absorbed by the body. It therefore provides few or no calories.

Complex carbohydrates are largely derived from wholegrain cereals such as wholemeal bread, oats, muesli and wholegrain rice. They are found in bran, wheat germ, barley, maize, buckwheat, semolina, oats, pasta, brown rice, potatoes, yams, manioc, taro, root vegetables, wholemeal bread, cereal bread, wholegrain cereals, high-fibre breakfast cereals, muesli, popis, beans and lentils. *glucose*: γλευκος (must, sweet new wine, sweet wine). In chemistry, it is the most common simple sugar, particularly in its D form (dextrose). The word was used by a committee of the French Academy of Sciences in 1838 to designate the sugar found in grapes, starch and honey, in reference to the etymology of the Greek (gleukos, sweet wine). Then there was the German chemist Emil Fischer who, after developing a step-by-step technique for synthesising sugars, established the structures of all known sugars between 1891 and 1894 by applying the principles of stereochemistry he had introduced. Glucose belongs to the family of hexoses, sugars containing six carbon atoms, divided into aldohexoses (allose, altrose, galactose, glucose, gulose, idose, mannose, talose) and ketohexoses (fructose, psicose, sorbose, tagatose). Emil Fischer's linear formula for the glucose molecule shows an unbranched chain of six carbon atoms. Carbon C-1 is part of an aldehyde group C(H)=O and the other five carbon atoms each carry a hydroxyl group OH. The four central carbon atoms are asymmetric, which gives glucose the ability to deflect the plane of incident polarised light: glucose is said to be optically active. Because it contains an aldehyde function, glucose is a reducing sugar. Glucose is a polar molecule thanks to its alcohol groups, which is why it is soluble in water and ethanol. It is also thermodegradable (caramelisation) and dialysable. In plants and some prokaryotes, glucose is the product of photosynthesis using water, carbon dioxide and light energy from the sun. In animals and fungi, glucose results from the depolymerisation of glycogen, a glucose polymer stored in the body. Industrially, glucose is obtained by enzymatic hydrolysis of starch. Various agricultural resources are used as sources of starch, including wheat, maize, rice and manioc[121] . Glucose is a ubiquitous fuel in biology. It is used as an energy source in most organisms, from bacteria to humans. All the cells in the human body are capable of using glucose to produce energy. This energy comes in the form of the ATP (Adenosine TriPhosphate) molecule and is produced in two stages: glycolysis and respiration in the mitochondria.

[121] "Glucose", *SCF,* consulted on 26/09/2023 (https://new.societechimiquedefrance.fr/produits/glucose/) p. 1-3.

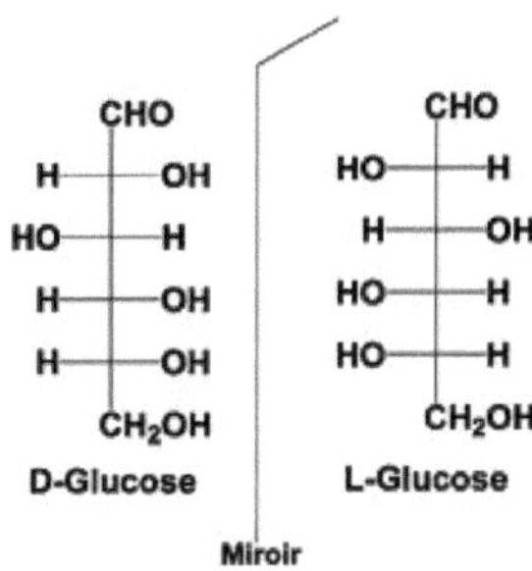

Linear formula for glucose by Emil Fischer glysine :

From the ancient Greek γλυκύς, glukos (sweet, soft) with the suffix -ine. Glycine (Gly or G) is an amino acid that is part of the composition of proteins. Like all amino acids, it has two functional groups, a carboxyl group (COOH) and an amine group (NH2). Its side chain is the simplest of all the amino acids, consisting of a single hydrogen atom (-H). It is not an essential amino acid, as it is synthesised from serine. As well as being a component of proteins, it is a neuromediator that acts on synapses and a precursor of numerous molecules (porphyrins).

In botany, Wisteria (Wistaria sinensis) is a climbing plant that can grow from 15 to 25 metres high. It is also known as Japanese wisteria or Chinese wisteria and, like alfalfa, is a member of the legume family.

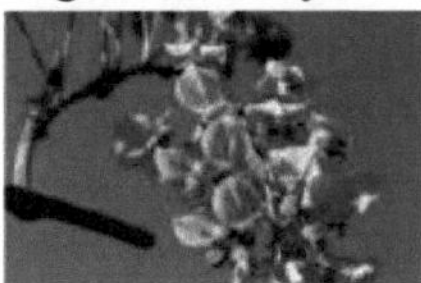

Clusters of wisteria.

It is an invasive creeper that can grow under roofs or fences. When pruned, it forms a small, dishevelled tree with a short, gnarled trunk. Its bark is grey and smooth. Its leaves are compound, between 20 and 30 cm long, and are light green in colour, with yellow on their own. In May-June, it flowers in clusters 20-70 cm long, usually bluish or white and highly fragrant. The fruit are green pods with brown pis, 15 to 25 cm long.[122]

night blindness: borrowed from the scientific Latin hemeralopia, composed of the Greek ἡμέρα, hemera, (day) and ωψ, ops (sight). It is the excessive difficulty in seeing when the light decreases (for example at dusk). It is also night blindness, i.e. the inability to perceive the small amounts of light that exist at night or during twilight, as well as during the day in artificially established

[122] Michel Caron, "Glycine: what is it?", Futura 02/05 (2023) p. 1-3.

darkness.
Haemorrhoid: From Latin haemorrhoida, borrowed from Ancient Greek αἱμορροΐς, haimorroïs, composed of αἷμα, haîma (blood), ῥόος, rhóos (current) and εἶδος, eîdos (type, aspect). This is the pathology of the anal canal in relation to the rectal (or haemorrhoidal) plexuses. These venous plexuses are anastomoses between the rectal veins located in the wall of the anal canal. This type of pathology is related to mechanical and vascular anomalies. They may be expressed by pain, bleeding or local discomfort. In other words, the veins in the anus and lower rectum are dilated. Constipation is the main cause, as it involves repeated pushing to pass faeces. Certain foods, such as meats, spicy foods, coffee, tea, colas and various alcoholic beverages, seem to encourage attacks. A diet low in fibre and insufficient hydration cause the stools to harden, making them difficult to pass.

Witch hazel leaves and bark contain tannins and flavonoids that are thought to increase the resistance of blood vessels. The rhizome of petit-houx contains numerous substances from the flavonoid family, which have vasoconstrictive (causing the walls of the blood vessels to contract) and vasculoprotective (protecting the walls of the blood vessels) properties. Chestnuts and horse chestnut bark contain æscine and æsculoside. These substances are thought to have a protective and stimulating effect on blood vessels. They also reduce inflammation. Blackcurrant leaves and berries contain anthocyanosides, substances with effects similar to those of vitamin P. The flowering tops of sweet clover contain flavonoids, which are thought to be responsible for its tonic and constrictive effects on blood vessels. They are thought to increase the resistance of blood vessels. Red vine leaves contain a large quantity of substances thought to have a protective and stimulating effect on veins and small blood vessels. Other plants used to relieve haemorrhoids include passionflower, white broth, ginger, ginkgo and climbing ivy. You can also use aloe vera gel and psyllium (or ispaghul) seeds.

However, people suffering from high blood pressure should consult their doctor before taking extracts of sweet clover, while those with liver problems should avoid sweet clover. Red vine contains resveratrol, which has an activity similar to that of hormones in the oestrogen family. Its use is not recommended for women with a personal or family history of breast or uterine cancer. For pregnant women, treatment of haemorrhoids should be limited to softening stools (with psyllium seeds, for example) and relieving pain locally (by applying creams or ointments to the anal region).

hepatitis: Ἡπατίτις, from ἦπαρ, ηπατος (liver). From Latin hepatitis. It is inflammation of the liver, of infectious, toxic or allergic origin. Viral hepatitis A is caused by a virus transmitted by ingestion. Hepatitis B is caused by a virus transmitted by blood, saliva or semen and hepatitis C is caused by a virus generally transmitted by blood transfusion.

herbaceous: From the Latin herbaceus (grass-coloured), from herba (grass). These are plants whose stems and branches do not produce wood and perish after a few months of vegetation. It is any perennial, annual or biennial plant that does not have a persistent woody stem above ground. It is a plant with flexible or soft stems, which are more or less buffer-like (not climbing, but can be erect), usually without lignin. Herbaceous plants are flowering plants, excluding algae, mosses and liverworts. They are found mainly in meadows, aquatic environments and gardens; a tomato shoot is a herbaceous plant, while a mango tree is a tree. Herbaceous plants also bear flowers and twigs, and sometimes collared leaves.

Homeopathy: From the ancient Greek δμοιος, hómoios (like, similar) and πάθος, pàthos (suffering, disease). Homeopathy or homœopathy is a pseudoscientific practice of non-conventional medicine according to which, it is possible to treat a patient by diluting very strongly substances which, if they were concentrated, would cause symptoms similar to those that the patient presents.

homeostasis: from the ancient Greek όμοιος, omoios, (similar) and στάσις stasis, (pause, stop).it is the capacity of an organism to maintain its internal physiological balance despite external constraints. In particular, homeostasis ensures the maintenance of body temperature, the number of blood cells in the blood and blood sugar levels. In the human body, the various homeostatic processes maintain water, oxygen, pH and blood sugar levels, as well as body temperature in different environments. In healthy organisms, these processes take place constantly and automatically. Hormones play a role in homeostasis. They are produced and secreted by endocrine glands, also known as ductless glands. The nervous system that regulates homeostasis is the hypothalamus, which reacts to the information received by sending messages via the nervous system. These messages are sent to the organs, which must then react to correct the situation. There are three components to homeostasis: the receptor, which detects the change occurring in the human body; the regulation centre, which processes the information received by the receptor and sends a response to the effector; and the effector, which brings about changes in the human body to encourage a return to equilibrium.

hormone: from ancient Greek ορμή, hormè (impulse) with the suffix -one. Substance produced by a gland. Hormones affect the development or functioning of an organ. There are a large number of hormones, which are essential for the body to function properly. The 5 hormones are: thyroid hormones, the guardians of metabolism; insulin, which controls blood sugar levels; serotonin, the messenger of happiness; cortisol, the stress hormone; and melatonin, the sleep hormone. Hormones are manufactured in small groups of specialised cells called pancreatic islets. The part of the pancreas that makes hormones is called the endocrine pancreas. The hormone of love, trust and connection, oxytocin, acts in several ways. Firstly, sexually, it enables men to eject sperm when they come, and women to have uterine spasms to help the sperm advance towards the egg. Dopamine is the hormone of immediate pleasure, in response to stimulation at a given moment. Serotonin, on the other hand, is a happiness hormone, stabilising mood over time. The 4 hormones of love are: testosterone, oestrogen, oxytocin (commonly known as the happiness hormone) and dopamine (a close cousin of the former, the reward hormone). In men, testosterone is predominant in the development of libido. This male sex hormone is also present in women, but in much smaller quantities. On the other hand, female sex hormones (progesterone and oestrogen) clearly influence desire during the cycle. Among the most important hormones in the body, "thyroid hormones, of which there are two, T3 (active hormone) and T4 (which converts to T3), have an effect on the metabolism of all the cells in the body. In the event of major stress, or of several stressful situations, the brain fills up with three hormones: adrenaline, noradrenaline and cortisol.

These three hormones play an important role in our mood and the well-being that follows.

hydragogue: From Ancient Greek ὑδραγωγός, hudragogos (that conducts or drains water). From Ancient Greek ὕδωρ, hÿdôr (water), ἀγωγή, agôgê (action of leading) or αγωγός , agôgos (who leads, who guides) derived from ἄγω , agô (to lead). It is a name applied to all agents capable of causing an evacuation of liquids such as: sudorifics, purgatives, diuretics. It is what has the property of evacuating serous liquids. Scammonium (Convolvulus scammonia) of the Convolvulaceae family is a true hydragogue which, as a drastic purgative, considerably increases secretion from the intestinal glands.

hydrate: From the ancient Greek ὕδωρ, hÿdôr (water) with the suffix -ate. In chemistry, hydrates are compounds formed by the union of water and another substance, a union usually resulting in a neutral body, such as certain crystallised salts. If the water is heavy water, where the hydrogen is in fact deuterium, we speak of deuterate rather than hydrate. So-called hydrated substances may contain water molecules chemically linked to the rest of the crystalline structure, or its constituent elements (H, O and/or OH) linked to the structure but separately. Clathrates are considered to be hydrates, for example methane hydrate. Compounds or minerals in which the water molecules are located in the cavities of the crystal lattice without a strong chemical bond are not considered to be hydrates; the water is simply absorbed, as in the case of clays. Oxides are precipitated from salts by alkaline bases in the hydrate state. Unlike hydrates, anhydrides are water-free compounds. Inorganic crystalline substances without water are called anhydrates or anhydrous. The best-known hydrate is soda ash, which is a decahydrated sodium carbonate. Hydrates are formed by hydration, generally during crystallisation from aqueous solutions. Hydrates rich in water of crystallisation can be dehydrated, for example by heating, so that either other hydrates containing less water of crystallisation are formed, or the anhydrous compound, colour changes often occur at the same time.

dropsy: Ancient Greek Ὑδρώπισις, dropsy, from υδρωψ, same meaning, which comes from ὕδωρ, water. In pathology, it refers to the accumulation of serosity, of non-inflammatory origin, in a natural cavity of the body or in cellular tissue. The term dropsy is a historical medical term used to designate any effusion of serosity in a natural body cavity or between elements of connective tissue. It could therefore be synonymous with oedema, generally affecting the lower limbs and more particularly the legs, ankles and feet. This condition occurs when the body's tissues begin to swell due to the accumulation of an organic liquid inside the cells. This is generally the liquid part of the blood, also known as blood serum. Blood, made up of fluids, salts and blood cells from various parts of the body, is transported by the blood vessels to the heart for purification. As a result, when there is an effusion of serosity or retention of fluids in the tissues and/or natural cavities of the body, the blood thickens and stagnates. This triggers swelling and the appearance of oedema.

Most of the time, dropsy as a disease referred to the main cause of generalised oedema, namely congestive heart failure. This disease is generally caused by excessive consumption of salty foods, prolonged sitting or standing, taking certain pharmaceutical products or irregular menstruation, congestive heart failure or venous insufficiency (commonly known as varicose veins), kidney failure, cirrhosis of the liver, pregnancy, calcifications, accidents or any obstruction in any part of the body. Grape seeds and red vine leaves help combat venous insufficiency. The condition can also be relieved by using extracts of the following plants: sage, cornflower, meadowsweet, garlic, artichoke, hawthorn, birch, borage, broom, cornflower, dandelion root, onion, horse chestnut, elderberry, raw cabbage leaves crushed with a rolling pin and used as a poultice to help reduce oedema. Cabbage is highly diuretic and depurative. It combats urine retention, oedema and dropsy, and helps eliminate excess water through sweat. Birch is highly effective against heart and kidney drops and oedema, and

is taken as an oral extract in 20 drops 4 times a day. Hawkweed has a very energetic diuretic action and is taken as an extract 4 times a day, 30 drops per dose. Elderberry extract needs 10 drops 5 times a day in a little water. Artichoke, known for its diuretic properties, can be taken daily in various forms: wine or tincture. To prepare the wine, macerate 40 dry leaves in 1 litre of white wine for 8 days. The decoction is then drunk in 2 small mustard glasses. To make the tincture, macerate 500g of cut, dried leaves in 1 litre of white brandy for 2 weeks. The liquid obtained is then filtered and stored in a bottle. To take, pour 2 teaspoons of this preparation into a little water and drink before meals[123] .
Hymenoptera: From the ancient Greek pteron, pteron (wing9 and 'umen, hymen (membrane), hence "membranous wing". The vast majority of Hymenoptera can be distinguished by their 2 pairs of membranous wings. Some are called pseudoparasitoids because they live inside the cocoons of spiders, eating their eggs. Hymenopteran parasitoids attack all orders of pterygote insects, but especially Lepidoptera. The most common are bees, wasps, ants and bumblebees. They range in size from 0.1 to 100 mm.
Hyperglycaemia: From the ancient Greek uper (above, above, superior), γλυκύς, glukús (sweet, sweet) and αίμα , haima (blood). This is an increase in blood sugar levels, above 1.20 g/l (> 10.0 mmol/L in most cases).
Hyperplasia: from the ancient Greek ὑπέρ, huper (on) and πλάσις, plasis (formation), It is sometimes synonymous with benign neoplasia or benign tumour. Hyperplasia is a medical term for hypergenesis; an abnormally large volume of an organic tissue or oragan due to an increase in the number of its cells (cell proliferation)[124] . This can lead to the hypertrophy of an organ. The most frequent clinical cases of hyperplasia or those likely to lead to hyperplasia are : benign prostatic hyperplasia (common after the age of 55)[125 126] ; Cushing's disease (chronic excess secretion of cortisol and secondarily of ACTH (adrenocorticotropic hormones), often induced by adrenocortical adenomas)[128;]

---

123 "Quand l'Hydropysie se soigne au naturel", Jardinier malin, Naure et Jardin, and Consulted on 18/06/ 2023 (https://www.jardiner-malin.fr/sante/soigner-hydropisie-plantes.html)1-3.
124 "Hyperplasia: MedlinePlus Medical Encyclopedia", consulted on 30/06/2023 (https://medlineplus.gov/ency/article/003441.htm)
125 "Prostate Enlargement: Benign Prostatic Hyperplasia", consulted on 30/06/2023 (https://www.niddk.nih.gov/health-information/urologic-diseases/prostate-problems/prostate- enlargement-benign-prostatic-hyperplasia).
126 "Cushing disease: MedlinePlus Medical Encyclopedia", Accessed on 30 /0672023 (https://medlineplus.gov/ency/article/000410.htm).

congenital adrenal hyperplasia (hereditary disorder of the adrenal gland)[127] ; endometrial hyperplasia (hyperproliferation of the endometrium).
in the uterus, often in response to unopposed oestrogen stimulation as part of polycystic ovary syndrome or exogenous hormone administration.
Hyperpyrexia: Πυρεξία, from πυρέσσειν, to have a fever, from πυρ, fever, fire. Nosology) Intense fever, characterised by an increase in body temperature above 41.5 °C.
Hypertension: From the Greek ὑπέρ, hyper (the highest degree, excess) and τείνω, teínô (to tend, unfold, move towards, relate to, concern). It is the rise in tension at the walls of a cavity when the pressure of the fluid it contains rises above its physiological values. It is caused by a multitude of factors, the effects of which accumulate over the years. The main ones are linked to age, heredity (especially in men) and lifestyle habits. Obesity, a sedentary lifestyle, smoking, alcohol abuse and stress all contribute to high blood pressure. It is a major risk factor for a number of diseases: heart and vascular disorders (angina, myocardial infarction and stroke); weakening of the arteries and increased risk of artery blockage through atherosclerosis; heart failure. By making the heart work harder, high blood pressure can lead to heart muscle exhaustion; kidney problems (renal failure) and eye problems (damage to the retina that can lead to loss of sight).
Blood pressure is made up of systolic and diastolic pressures, measured in millimetres of mercury, or mmHg. Systolic pressure is the pressure of the blood when the heart contracts and sends blood into the arteries. Diastolic pressure is the pressure that continues to be exerted on the arteries between each contraction. At this point, the heart relaxes and regains its volume, allowing the heart chambers to fill with blood. This pressure tends to increase with age, but after the age of sixty it gradually decreases as the body's blood vessels weaken. So when we talk about a blood pressure of 120/80, 120 corresponds to systolic pressure and 80 to diastolic pressure. One of the best natural remedies for lowering blood pressure is garlic. Rich in selenium, a trace element with antioxidant properties, in addition to its effects on high blood pressure, it reduces levels of bad cholesterol and acts against atherosclerosis. Lavender, fennel and camomile have a proven positive effect on the potassium channel, which relaxes the blood vessels, thereby reducing blood pressure; green and black tea have a similar effect on the potassium channel. Raw or lightly cooked

[127] "Congenital adrenal hyperplasia: MedlinePlus Medical Encyclopedia", Accessed on 30/0672023 (https://medlineplus.gov/ency/article/000411.htm).

broccoli is rich in calcium, magnesium, potassium and flavonoids, making it a protective food against coronary heart disease, which can be caused by high blood pressure[128] Sweet potatoes are among the starches with the lowest glycemic index and are rich in potassium, calcium and magnesium; cocoa is rich in flavonoids, which help the body cope better with stress (a frequent cause of high blood pressure) and protect against heart disease; it is also rich in magnesium and potassium; turmeric, an anti-cancer, anti-inflammatory and risk reducer for cardiovascular disease, is almost a miracle spice, with anti-coagulant and anti-inflammatory properties; bananas contain the trio of minerals that protect the cardiovascular system, such as magnesium, potassium and calcium, as well as being rich in fibre, antioxidants and vitamins B and C; artichokes contain good quantities of potassium and are also very good for the liver thanks to its
diuretic properties that help eliminate excess fluids in the body, thereby lowering blood pressure. Tomatoes have a high antioxidant capacity, contain numerous vitamins and amino acids and, above all, potassium, which prevents blood pressure from rising[129] .

Hypoglycaemia: From the Greek ύπο, hypo (below, small amount, decrease, insufficiency), γλυκύς glukús (sweet, sugary) and αίμα haîma (blood). This is the lowering of blood glucose concentration below 3.6 mmol/L or less than 0.6g/L, leading to various general disorders (weakness, sweating, craving, syncope). It is generally caused by excessive consumption of simple sugars, sugary foods between meals, meals low in fibre and complex sugars, etc. Reactive hypoglycaemia results in symptoms such as tiredness and paleness, dizziness, hunger and craving for sweet foods, tremors, headaches, blurred vision and sweating. To remedy hypoglycaemia, you can use natural remedies such as Black Mulberry, which combats diabetes, pancreatic insufficiency and hypoglycaemia. Bilberry promotes sugar assimilation and helps regulate insulin levels. Gymnena (gymnema sylvestris) is effective in maintaining optimal blood glucose levels thanks to its gymnemic acid, which helps to reduce sugar absorption and improve insulin secretion. Berberine, a molecule extracted from Berberis vulgaris and Berberis aristata, is a plant alkaloid which reduces fasting

---

[128] Houston MC, Harper KJ, Potassium, magnesium, and calcium: their role in both the cause and treatment of hypertension, J Clin Hypertens (Greenwich), 2/10/7 (2008) p. 3-11.

[129] "10 aliments pour faire baisser sa tension. Paseport Santé, consulted on 20/06/2023
(https://www.passeportsante.net/fr/Actualites/Dossiers/DossierComplexe.aspx?doc=10-aliments- pour-faire-baisser-sa-tension) 1-4.

and post-meal glycaemia, glycated haemoglobin, plasma insulin levels and cholesterol. It also acts on and protects the activity of the pancreatic beta cells responsible for insulin production. It is a truly effective molecule for people suffering from diabetes. Ginseng is an extraordinary adaptogenic plant which, in addition to its effect on glucose, adapts to different stresses. Garlic is an antibiotic, an antiseptic and a regulator of hyperglycaemia. Cinnamon has anti-diabetic properties and regulates blood sugar levels by facilitating the work of insulin[130] .

hyperthermia: Hyperthermia is a rise in body temperature caused by a disturbance in thermoregulation. It is induced by an increase in thermogenesis or a decrease in thermolysis, following intense physical exercise or heat stroke.

infusion: From the Latin infusio (to infuse), from infundere (to pour into). This is the process of allowing substances to infuse in a liquid for varying lengths of time in order to extract their soluble principles. It is also the drink resulting from the dissolution of the active principles of a plant, obtained by pouring boiling water over the plant or part or extracts of the plant.

idiosyncrasy: From Ancient Greek ιδιοσυγκρασία / idiosunkrasia (the same, oneself, peculiar temperament), from 'ίδιος / ídios (proper, peculiar), σύν / sún (with), and κρασις / krâsis (mixture). It is the particular behaviour, the psychic personality 1, peculiar to an individual. In medicine, it is the particular disposition by virtue of which each individual reacts in a way peculiar to him to an external agent, physical or chemical, and to the influences of the various agents that affect his organs. It is also the body's particular disposition to react in an unusual way to a drug or substance.

immunity: Latin immunitas, from the Latin word immunis, (exempt). This is the property possessed by certain living beings of not being able to contract again, or of contracting without seriousness, a disease they have already had or against which they have been vaccinated. It is also the state of an organism that is resistant to infection by a micro-organism or to the toxic effects of an antigenic substance, whether of microbial origin or not. Immunity can be specific or non-specific, innate or acquired, humoral, cellular or mixed. To protect itself, the human body has 2 types of defence mechanism: innate immunity and adaptive immunity. Innate immunity enables the body to defend itself against infectious agents immediately. Adaptive immunity, on the other hand, provides protection that comes later, but lasts longer.

---

[130] "Anti-diabetes plants: lowering blood sugar levels with plants", Mes bienfaits, consulted on 20/06/2023 (https://www.mesbienfaits.com/plantes-diabete-glycemie/) p. 1-4.

insecticide: From insect by adding the suffix - cide, from the Latin caedere (to kill). It is a substance that destroys insects. Insecticides are active substances or plant protection preparations with the property of killing insects, their larvae and/or their eggs. They belong to the family of pesticides, which in turn belong to the family of biocides. The generic term insecticide also includes pesticides designed to combat arthropods that are not insects (e.g. spiders or mites such as ticks), as well as repellents. A distinction is made between products that act by contact, systemic products, and intermediate-mode products, known as translaminar products.

larvicide: From the Latin larva (appearance, ghost) and occidere (to kill, eliminate). It refers to a product or preparation that has the property of killing larvae. *leucorrhoea*: From the ancient Greek λευκός, leukos (white) and ρέω, rhéô (to flow). A leucorrhoea, or white discharge, is a more or less abundant vaginal discharge, white or tinted, odorous or not, fluid or thick. It may be physiological or indicate the presence of a genital infection[131] Secretions do not cause irritation, are odourless and depend on hormones. They appear at puberty and disappear at the menopause[132] . They mainly come from cervical mucus, vaginal desquamation, vaginal transudate from the venous plexuses, and secretions from the vulval glands (Skene's and Bartholin's glands). Non-menopausal adult women produce between 1ml and 4ml per day, with variations depending on age, the menstrual cycle, whether they are taking hormones and sexual stimulation[133] [134] In menopausal women, hormonal deficiency leads to atrophy and changes in the flora, giving the appearance of senile vaginitis[136] . Secretions may be white, caseous, purulent, green or greyish, and associated with pruritus, burning or a musty odour. Most often, the cause is infectious: vulvitis, vaginitis, cervicitis, endometritis or salpingitis. The agents responsible are either bacteria (Gardnerella vaginalis, gonococcus, chlamydia, mycoplasma), fungi (Candida Albicans) or parasites (Trichomonas vaginalis). In lower genital infections, yeasts, Trichomonas and common germs are more often found. Treatment of the infection will depend on the causative agent. Excessive

[131] Éditions Larousse, "Leucorrhée ou perte blanche ou perte vaginale - LAROUSSE", consulted on 29/06/ 2023 (https://www.larousse.fr/encyclopedie/medical/leucorrh%C3%A9e/14198).

[132] "Les ennuis et maladies génicologiques : les pertes blanches", consulted on 29/06/2023 (http://www.cngof.fr/maladies/343-les-pertes-blanches).

[133] J. -M. Bohbot, "Les sécrétions vaginales", Pelvi-périnéologie, Volume 3, Issue 1, 3 (2008) p. 19-24, March 2008.

[134] "Female genital infections. Leucorrhoea", Accessed on 29/06/2023 (http://www.cngof.net/E-book/GO-2016/CH-28.htm).

intimate hygiene using detergent soaps can encourage these infections by destroying the vaginal ecosystem. In rare cases, it may be indicative of cervical cancer, and exceptionally may be caused by the presence of an intravaginal foreign body.

lepidoptera: From the Latin lepidoptera, itself from the ancient Greek λεπίς, lepís (scale) and πτερόν , pterón (wing). They are an order of holometabolous insects whose adult form (or imago) is commonly called a butterfly, whose larva is called a caterpillar, and whose nymph is called a chrysalis. There are more than 257 species of day and 5200 species of night lepidopterans. Its body is made up of three parts: the head, the thorax and the abdomen.

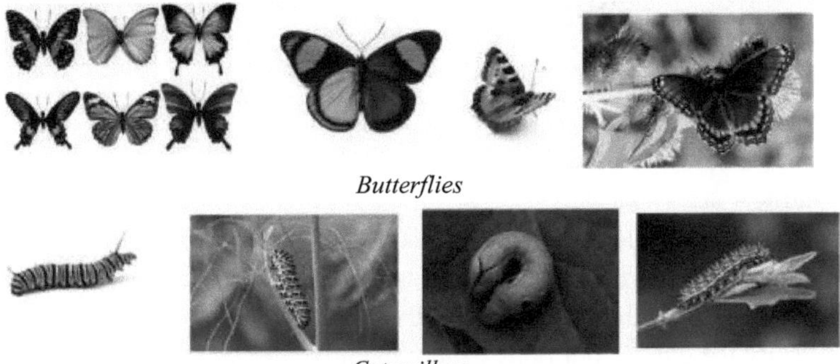

Butterflies

Caterpillars

The *nymph* is the intermediate stage of development between the larva and the imago during metamorphosis, particularly in holometabolous insects. The stage The nymphal stage begins with the moult of a larva into a nymph (nymphal moult or pupation) and ends with the moult of the nymph into an imago (imaginal moult or adult moult). One of the characteristics of the nymph is that it does not feed (its mouth parts and digestive tract also undergo metamorphosis) and that it lives on its reserves.

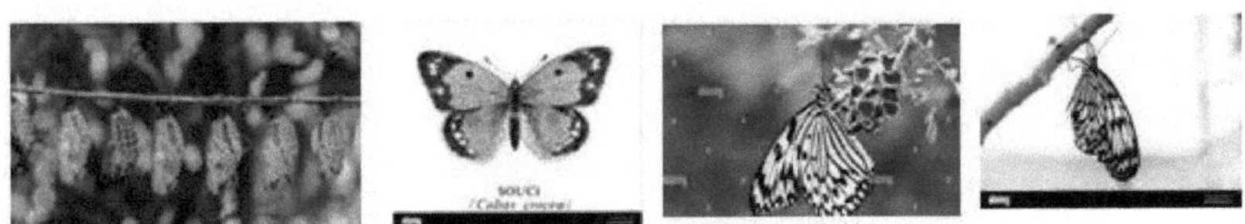

butterfly nymphs

The pupa of Lepidoptera is often called the chrysalis. In Diptera, the equivalent of the pupa is the pupa, with the difference that the pupa remains inside the last larval cuticle (absence of pupal exuviation). In some species, the nymph is protected by a concon.

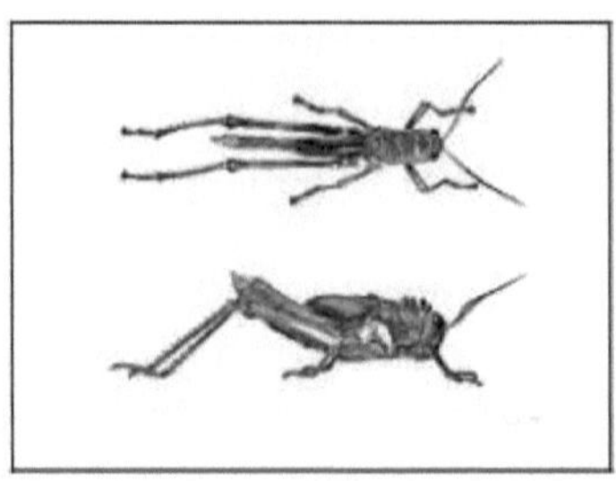

Tropidacris cristata nymph

The word nymph is sometimes used (especially in translations of foreign literature) to designate the immature forms (larvae) of hemimetabolic insects with wing outlines (as in termites, locusts and grasshoppers, in which the wings appear gradually), but which, in this case, feed.

liposoluble: from the Greek lipos (fat) and the Latin solubilis (to dissolve). In chemistry, a substance that is soluble in lipids or fats, for example vitamins A, D, E and K.

lysine: From the ancient Greek lusis (solution, dissolution) and -ine; probably influenced by the German lysin. This is an amino acid, a constituent of proteins, which cannot be synthesised by the body and is essential for growth. It must be provided by the diet, as our body cannot manufacture it. This acid is used by the body in the synthesis of proteins, but also as a source of energy when necessary. It promotes the intestinal absorption of calcium and can therefore help prevent osteoporosis. Lysine also has antiviral activity, particularly in cases of herpes, which is responsible for the appearance of cold sores. It can also help reduce fatigue. It is found in meat (beef, chicken, veal, pork, turkey), fish, eggs and dairy products, as well as legumes, particularly soya. It is also present in corn and corn products. Amino acids ensure that the body functions properly and has the energy it needs to grow, develop and maintain muscles and organs. They also enable the immune system to function properly. Its chemical formula is C6H14N2O2.

maceration: From the Latin maceratio (maceration, soaking), from macero (macerate, soak). This is the operation of leaving a solid body in a liquid or humid medium to extract certain active or nutritive principles from the body or to obtain a change in the body; the state of a body subjected to this action.

microbiota: From the Greek μικρός, mikrós or σμικρός, smikrós (small, of little importance, weak, which lasts a short time) and βιωτός biôtós, from βιόω, bióô (to live, to live). It refers to all the populations of microorganisms that colonise a particular environment: intestinal microbiota, faecal microbiota, skin microbiota, oral microbiota. A microbiota includes not only prokaryotes (bacteria and archaea) but also fungi, protozoa and, by extension, viruses. The intestinal microbiota is the most important of these, with around 1013 microorganisms, which is the same order of magnitude as the number of cells that make up the human body, weighing in at around 1.5 kilos.

medicament : From Latin *medicamentum* (same meaning), made from *medicare* (to give remedies), derived from Greek μηδος (care). It is an active principle, a substance of chemical or natural origin characterised by a precise curative or preventive mechanism of action in the body. In France, the Public Health Code (article L.5111-1) defines a medicinal product as follows: "*any substance or composition presented as having curative or preventive properties with regard to human or animal diseases, as well as any substance or composition which may be used in or administered to humans or animals, with a view to establishing a medical diagnosis or to restoring, correcting or modifying their physiological functions by exerting a pharmacological, immunological or metabolic action*"[135] . Medicines, as defined, are subject to highly controlled and monitored manufacturing, distribution and administration standards. Medicinal products contains: an *active ingredient*, a substance of chemical or natural origin with a specific curative or preventive action in the body; *excipients*, substances of chemical or natural origin which facilitate the use of the medicine but have no curative or preventive effect. There are several categories of medicines, including: *proprietary medicinal products*, which are industrially manufactured medicines used by pharmaceutical companies. Before they can be dispensed to patients, they must obtain a marketing authorisation (MA). The same proprietary medicinal product may have a different brand name in different countries. The international non-proprietary name (INN) is used to give a unique designation for the active substance it contains; magistral, hospital or officinal preparations, which are most often made by a pharmacy for the specific needs of one or more patients (dispensary for magistral and officinal preparations or pharmacy for internal use in a health establishment for magistral and hospital preparations). These pharmaceutical preparations and specialities come in a variety of pharmaceutical forms: tablets, oral solutions, injectable solutions and others.

[135] Ministère de la Santé et de la Prévention (MSP), "Qu'est-ce qu'un médicament", *MSP* 16/04 (2022) p. 1.

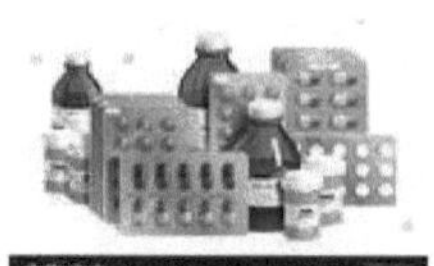
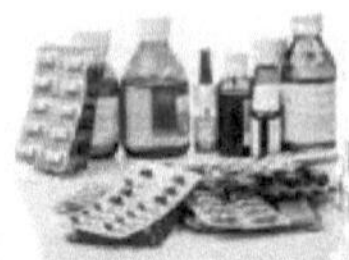
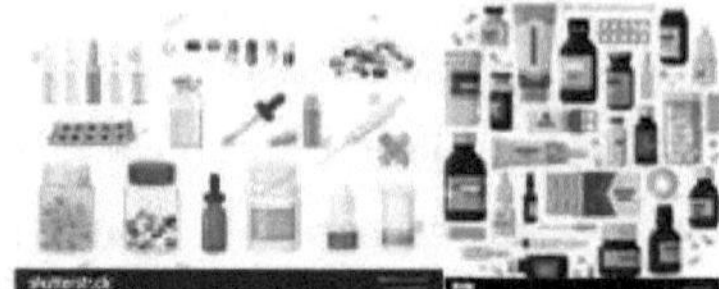
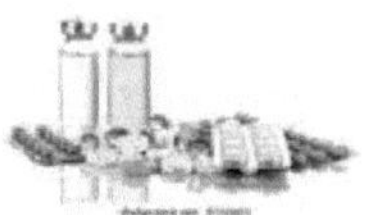

microcytic: From the Greek *mikros* (small) and *kutos* (cavity, cell). Pertaining to microcytosis, which refers to the presence of small red blood cells in the blood. Microcytosis observed on a blood smear (examination of the blood under a microscope) is reported to be slight to ++++ (4 plus). This observation is useful in the differential diagnosis of anaemias, which are divided according to the size of the red blood cells into microcytic, normocytic or macrocytic anaemia. A GMV (mean corpuscular volume) below the norm is another way of indicating microcytosis. The most common causes of microcytic anaemia are iron deficiency, a very prolonged inflammatory state, chronic bleeding (digestive, uterine) or certain genetic defects in haemoglobin production (thalassaemia). There are five main causes of microcytic anaemia: thalassaemia, chronic anaemia, iron deficiency, lead poisoning and congenital sideroblastic anaemia.
moxibustion: From moxa which comes from the Japanese *mogusa* (burning herbs) and the Latin radical bustio which is in com-bustio (combustion), burning herbs. It is the method of cauterisation or ustion specific to the various substances with which moxas can be made.
neurasthenia: Greek νευρον, neûron (nerve) and ασθένεια, asthéneia (weakness, illness). Neurasthenia, also referred to medically as chronic fatigue syndrome, is a psychopathological term first used by George Miller Beard in 1869[136] to refer to a condition whose symptoms include fatigue, anxiety, headaches, neuralgia, a loss of zest for life and decreased activity (dejection). The symptoms are similar to those of a viral-type illness, with adenopathy, extreme fatigue, fever and upper respiratory symptoms. The initial syndrome resolves but seems to trigger severe and prolonged fatigue, which disrupts daily activities and is generally aggravated by exertion, which is not relieved by rest. Patients often also have sleep and cognitive problems, such as memory problems, 'foggy thinking', hypersomnolence and a feeling of having had a non-restorative sleep. Important general characteristics are diffuse pain and sleep problems. In phytotherapy,

[136] G. Beard, "Neurasthenia, or nervous exhaustion", The Boston Medical and Surgical Journal, (1869) p. 217-221.

olantes are used to relieve fatigue: ginseng, particularly in herbal tea, eleutherococcus (Siberian ginseng), caffeine-based plants (coffee seeds, guarana, tea or maté leaves, kolatian nuts); lemon balm for restful sleep; ginseng during convalescence; eleutherococcus against overwork; ginger against sexual weakness.

nutirment: From the Latin *nutrimentum* (food). It is an organic and mineral compound that can be assimilated by a living organism and is vital for its development and maintenance. It is also a substance supplied by food and used by the body for its construction and functioning. *Nutrients* provide the body with the energy and materials it needs to cover its expenses and ensure cell renewal. The main *nutrients* are found in food in the form of macromolecules, which are then broken down by the digestive system to be assimilated. Water is the most important *nutrient*, accounting for 60% of our total intake. It is a word introduced recently to designate substances that can nourish without passing through the stomach and undergoing digestive action; such as albumin, broths and osmazoa.

Also known as nutrients, nutrients are molecules derived from food and mainly produced by the digestive process. When these nutrients are assimilated by the body, we speak of nutrition. Nutrients are essential for meeting the various physiological needs of the human body, including bone development and growth. Nutrients perform a variety of functions, such as providing energy, regulating metabolism and maintaining tissues. There are: -Macronutrients: proteins, which play a structural role, particularly in tissue renewal; carbohydrates, which are the body's energy fuel; lipids, which also play a structural role and store energy.

-Micronutrients: vitamins, minerals and trace elements that the body cannot synthesise and which are essential for our body to function properly.

-Mesonutrients: these are the "health" molecules present in food which have a protective role (antioxidants, carotenoids, polyphenols, omega 3, etc.).

Essential nutrients are those that are essential for the body to function properly, in particular: fatty acids (omega-3, omega-6), amino acids, vitamins (vitamin A, group B vitamins, vitamin C, vitamins D, E and K), minerals (sodium, potassium, calcium, iron, zinc, phosphorus, magnesium, iodine, selenium, etc.).

Recommended daily allowances (RDAs) for macronutrients vary according to each individual's build, age, sex and physical activity. Overall, an adult's total nutritional intake should be 45-50% carbohydrate, 15% protein and 30-35% fat.

On average: men aged 20 to 40 need 2,700 calories; men aged 41 to 60 need 2,500 calories; women aged 20 to 40 need 2,200 calories; women aged 41 to 60 need 2,000 calories.

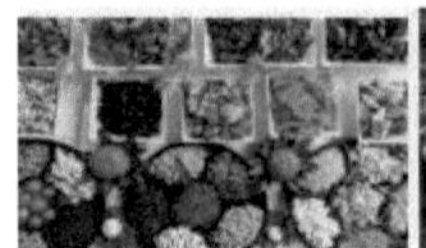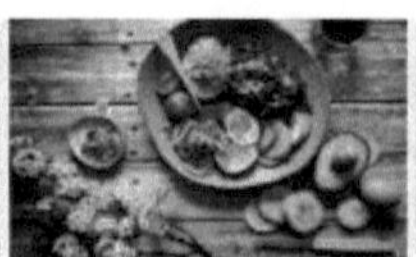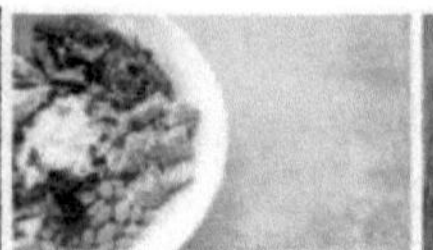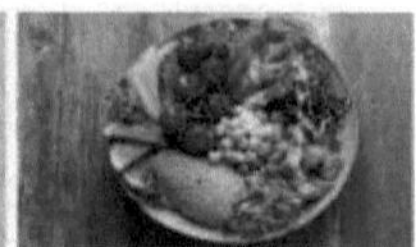

Carbohydrates are found in cereal products, pulses and dairy products. Proteins are found in eggs, meat, fish, dairy products, nuts and seeds. Good fats are found in avocado, olive oil, rapeseed oil, oily fish (mackerel, sardines, salmon, herring), almonds and walnuts. Vitamins and minerals are found mainly in plants (fruit and vegetables), meat, fish and shellfish[139] . Nutritional deficiencies are accompanied by a weakened immune system, fatigue, sleep disorders, muscle cramps, hair loss, concentration problems and lack of motivation.

oblong: From the Latin oblongus (elongated, oblong). A shape that is longer than it is wide and rounded at both ends. In geometry, it refers to a figure that is longer than it is wide. In botany, the term refers to the oblong leaves of a plant whose blade is longer than wide and rounded at the ends.

oboval: from ob-, (idea of facing, and also of reversal). From Sanskrit abhi, corresponding to the Gothic iup, and from Latin ovalis, from ovum (egg). In botany, this refers to a plant or part of a plant that has an inverted oval shape, i.e. the upper part is larger than the lower part.

139

Julie Giorgetta, "Nutrient: definition, examples, role, essentials", *Le journal de Femmes* Santé 15/04 (2022) p.

ocimene: Named after one of the plants that contains it, basil or Ocimum basilicum. It is a fragrant monoterpene organic compound of which there are several isomers. Its molecular formula is C10H16. It has four closely related isomers that differ in the location of their unsaturations. It is also a component of many essential oils derived from plants. This molecule is found in various plants with properties and stabilities that prevent its oxidation. It is used in oils and perfumes for its scent. This molecule is also known as a pheromone.

oxytocin: from the ancient Greek ώκύς, ocy for ôkus (quick), and from tocine for τόκος, tokos (childbirth). In biochemistry, it is a hormone secreted by the posterior lobe of the pituitary gland, which excites the contraction of the uterus at the time of childbirth and which also acts on the contraction of the alveoli and milk ducts of the mammary gland, resulting in the secretion of milk. It binds to its own receptors in the myometrium, the number of which increases as pregnancy approaches term. Synthetically produced oxytocin is a drug that prevents post-partum haemorrhage by helping the uterus to contract. It is administered to the mother by intravenous or intramuscular injection during or immediately after the birth of the child. Oxytocin is also considered to be the love hormone that invades at the moment of orgasm[140.] It is involved in sexual reproduction, particularly during and after childbirth[141] . It is released in large quantities (6x more in the first 3

[140] Netgen, "Oxytocin: the hormone of love, trust and the marital and social bond", *Swiss Medical Journal,* Accessed 30/06/ 2023 (https://www.revmed.ch/revue-medicale-suisse/2012/revue-medicale-suisse-333/l-ocytocine- hormone-of-love-of-confidence-and-of-marital-and-social-bonding).

[141] L.Jennifer et als, "Oxytocin/Vasopressin-Related Peptides Have an Ancient Role in Reproductive Behavior" Science (2012) 338(6106):540-3. PMID 23112335.

months of pregnancy and up to 86x more at birth)[137] after distension of the cervix and uterus during labour, which facilitates birth, and after stimulation of the nipples or breastfeeding. It plays an important role in a range of behaviours, such as orgasm, social recognition, empathy, anxiety and maternal behaviour, hence its nickname of "pleasure hormone", "happiness hormone"[138] , or "attachment hormone" between mother and child. In certain situations, oxytocin could also induce "radical" or even violent behaviour in defence of the group, for example when faced with a third party refusing to cooperate. It would then become a source of defensive (rather than offensive) aggression[139] . Oxytocin is mainly synthesised by the brain, but it is also secreted by many cell types other than those of the nervous system. Synthesis is continuous, but with periods of greater activity.

odontalgia: From the Greek οδος, 'odos (tooth) and άλγος, algos (pain). This is toothache. Odontalgia is often the consequence of damage to a tooth or the surrounding tissues (gums, tongue, jaws, etc.). It can also be caused by hypersensitivity of the tooth: pain on contact with hot or cold (air passing into the mouth, cold water, hot foods, but also sweet or acidic foods); a painful sensation on touch (sensitivity when brushing the teeth). It can also be triggered by the impact between several teeth. Teeth are made up of enamel, dentin and

---

[137] Marcel Hibert, *Oxytocin, my love* 9 (2021) 251 p.

[138] Other hormones such as testosterone, known as the "desire hormone", prolactin, which has a libidinal effect, and luiberin, which triggers mating, are also thought to play a role in the creation of the amorous state. Source: Jean-Didier Vincent, Biologie des passions, Odile Jacob, (1999) p. 242.

[139] Viviane Thivent, "Oxytocin or the hormone of sacrifice?", Biology and Health, 17/06 (2010) p.
1.

pulp. One of the main causes is tooth decay. This is caused by microbial growth in the enamel and dentine. It leads to inflammation of the tooth pulp. The pain can range from increased sensitivity of the tooth to severe spontaneous pain (toothache), to acute pain of great intensity in the area where the decay is located. It can extend as far as the ears, jaws or sinuses. The same type of pain can be caused by dental trauma, such as a crack, abrasion or fracture. It can also be caused by a chronic infection of the enamel, dentine or pulp of the tooth, an abscess of the gum or damage to other tooth-supporting tissue, such as periodontitis. It may also be the result of a more distant infection: otitis, eye disease, shingles, sinusitis; or of teething: baby teeth in childhood, then permanent teeth, with wisdom teeth often causing severe radiating pain. Symptoms include swollen gums, gum pain, bleeding, headaches, fever, bad breath and a bad taste in the mouth[140] .

oleic: From the Latin oleum (oil) with the suffix -ic. Oleic acid is a monounsaturated fatty acid from the omega-9 family. It is mainly found in vegetable oils such as olive oil, avocado oil, safflower oil and canola oil. It makes up 55% to 80% of the fatty acids in olive oil. Highly present in the human body, it protects the cardiovascular system and reduces cholesterol. Its structure is C18H34O2.

Trace element: from the Greek oligos (small, not abundant) is defined as an entity present in very small quantities in our bodies. In biology, it is a mineral element present in very small quantities (traces) in living organisms and essential to their functioning: chromium (Cr), cobalt (Co), copper (Cu), tin (Sn), fluorine (F), manganese (Mn), molybdenum (Mo), selenium (Se), silicon (Si), vanadium (V) and zinc (Zn). They are used in the composition of enzymes or are necessary for their activation. Along with silver, copper and selenium, gold is one of the trace elements most commonly prescribed by doctors to treat fatigue, high blood pressure, psoriasis, arthritis and Raynaud's disease. The 10 trace elements that boost health[141] :

-Gold to fight viruses. Gold is generally used by oligotherapists in synergy with copper and silver to broaden its field of action. This mineral, which is not naturally present in the body, has renowned anti-infectious properties. Along with silver, copper and selenium, it is one of the trace elements most commonly prescribed by doctors to treat fatigue, high blood pressure, psoriasis, arthritis and Raynaud's disease.

-Calcium strengthens bones, helps build bone and teeth structure, and helps

---

[140] Sophie Zimmermann, "L'odontalgie: qu'est-ce que c'est?", Passeport Santé 20/12 (2022) 1-5.

Sophie Laurent, "Les 10 oligo-éléments qui boostent la santé", *Femme Actuelle* 07/02 (2022) p.1-4.

prevent cardiovascular disease, colon cancer and osteoporosis. This trace element is also involved in the coagulation process and promotes muscle contraction. Its daily intake of around 900 mg for adults is even more important for the elderly and pregnant women. Calcium is also found in dairy products, dates, dried beans and egg yolks.

-Cobalt relieves migraines and helps to combat vascular pathologies such as arterial hypertension and Raynaud's disease. It also has anti-fatigue properties. It is present in herring, mackerel, liver, kidneys, seafood and milk.

-Copper stimulates the immune system. It is an all-purpose trace element. It fights infections, inflammation, viruses and fatigue thanks to its immunogenic power, triggering the production of antibodies, red blood cells, elastin and collagen. It is recommended for viral infections and rheumatic conditions. It is found in shellfish, chocolate, liver, starchy foods and red wine.

-Fluoride promotes beautiful teeth thanks to the properties of this metalloid on bones, to prevent and treat osteoporosis. It is present in fish, tea, seaweed, mineral water, pineapple, asparagus and many other foods.

-Iron protects against anaemia, being one of the major constituents of haemoglobin. As such, it plays a major role in the cell oxygenation mechanism. This is why it is particularly used in cases of fatigue or intense muscular effort. Iron deficiencies are relatively common, particularly during pregnancy, as the daily requirements are not adequately covered by the modern diet. Iron is present in red meat, green vegetables, dairy products and fruit. It should be noted that certain other foods reduce the absorption of this mineral, such as coffee, bran and tea.

- Silver is an excellent antiviral agent. It combats fatigue, prevents viral infections and treats certain dermatological conditions such as shingles and acne thanks to its bactericidal properties. It is a trace element that is mostly associated with other minerals such as gold and copper.

-Chromium is effective against excess sugar. It is an essential element in the process of metabolising lipids and carbohydrates. It is a very important mineral for preventing cardiovascular disease, diabetes and obesity. It is found in liver, egg yolk, brewer's yeast, seafood and black tea.

-Selenium combats ageing. As a cellular antioxidant, it plays a preventive role in many cancers. It has a direct effect on the central nervous system, combating age-related macular degeneration and Alzheimer's disease. It is particularly present in meat, eggs, fish and cereals.

- Iodine relieves thyroid problems. It is particularly effective in the treatment of thyroid disorders and as a dietary supplement in cases of thyroid insufficiency. It is found in shellfish, fish, green beans, dairy products and soya.

ophthalmic: Greek οφθαλμός, ophtalmós (eye), suffix -ique: Having to do with the eye, e.g. ophthalmic migraine, often preceded by precursor signs: fatigue, depression or irritability, digestive disorders; the ophthalmic artery, which is a branch of the internal carotid artery that supplies the eye and orbit.
orbicularis: From the Latin orbicularis, from orbiculus (small circle), diminutive of orbis (circle). Said of something that has the shape of an orb, a sphere or a circle. Example: the orbicularis muscle is the ring-shaped muscle located around a natural orifice of the face, used to close this orifice by contraction. The eye orbicularis muscle (Musculus orbicularis oculi in Latin) or eyelid orbicularis muscle is a muscle that forms an elliptical area around the eyelids and extends in a thin layer over the eyelids themselves. It is traditionally divided into three parts: palpebral, orbital and lacrimal. The orbicularis muscle of the mouth (Musculus orbicularis oris in Latin) or orbicularis muscle of the lips is made up of four sections of muscle around the mouth opening, which above all forms the framework of the lips. The kiss is the anatomical superposition of these sections of orbicularis oris muscle in a state of contraction, which is why this muscle is commonly referred to as the "kissing muscle".
orthodiptera: from the Greek orqoV, orthos (straight) and pteron, pteron (wing*)*. The orthopterans or Orthoptera are an order of insects characterised by wings aligned with the body: grasshoppers, crickets, locusts and crickets. They have long hind legs adapted for jumping and two pairs of wings carried along the back. Body length varies between 5 mm and 15 cm, depending on the species. Colours also vary from species to species, particularly in the
locusts. Crickets have thick antennae that are shorter than their bodies. They account for almost half of the species in the

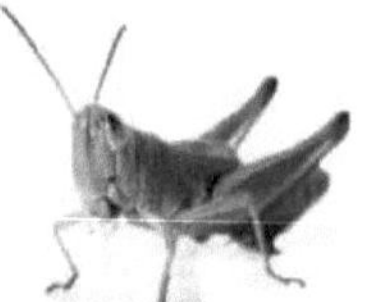 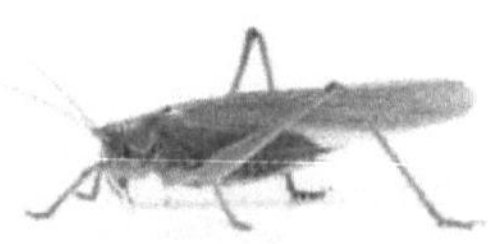 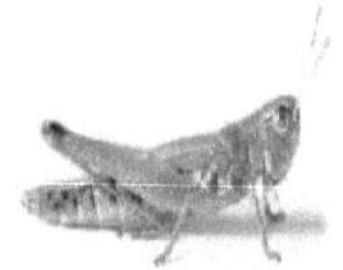

Grasshoppers with thin, long antennae

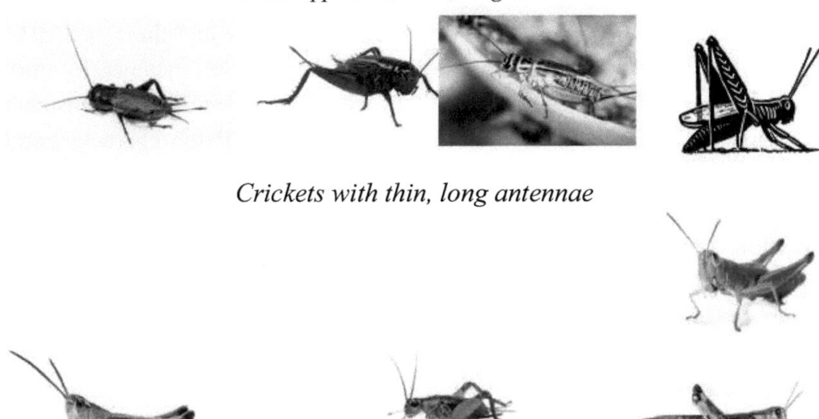

Crickets with thin, long antennae

Locusts

Grasshoppers and crickets have long, slender antennae. Unlike grasshoppers, crickets have hind legs set apart from the rest of the body and are never green in colour. Orthopterans can make sounds called stridulations. This "song", which is specific to each species, plays a role in forming pairs for reproduction. For most grasshoppers and crickets, only the males make these sounds by rubbing two wings together. Locusts rub their hind legs against their wings.

oside: From ancient Greek -ωσις , -õsis, (state, abnormal condition or action), from -όω (- óõ) verbal root and -σις, -sis. -ose. This is a hydrolysable carbohydrate, i.e. capable of giving rise to one or more oses by hydrolysis. Lactose and maltose are osides. In chemistry, this is the generic name given to non-hydrolysable organic substances with a reducing group, aldehyde or ketone, and more than two alcoholic functions. They are divided into trioses, tetroses, pentoses, hexoses and heptoses, depending on whether they contain 3, 4, 5, 6 or 7 carbon atoms. They are also divided into aldoses and ketoses depending on whether they have aldehyde or ketone functions. In biochemistry, it is a chemical compound with the general formula CnH2nOn, made up of a chain of carbon atoms each bearing an alcohol function (-OH), except for one which bears a carbonyl function (-CO-). The two best-known oses are glucose and fructose.

osteoporosis: From the Greek οστέον, osteon (bone) and πόρος, póros (passage, way of communication, conduit or passage for humours, secretions, respiration). It is a bone pathology that consists of the rarefaction of the protein framework of the bone and the decrease in its mineral density with enlargement of the medullary cavities and spaces. The bones become brittle and there is a risk of fractures. It usually occurs in women after the menopause, or generally during prolonged corticosteroid treatment, in various pathological circumstances, particularly endocrine. It is also the alteration of the skeleton characterised by the progressive rarefaction of bone tissue due to decalcification, which has the effect of weakening the bones. Bone fragility leads to fractures, which are the main clinical manifestation of the disease. The three main fractures involve the neck of the femur, the vertebrae and the distal part of the radius. Fracture loss is assessed by bone densitometry, which analyses bone mineral density (BMD). The reference measurement is called the T-score. If the measurement is greater than -1, the bone density is normal; if it is between -2.5 and -, it is a case of brittle bone or osteopenia; if it is less than or equal to -2.5, it is osteoporosis; if it is less than or equal to -2.5 with fracture(s), it is severe osteoporosis.[145]

Decoctions, infusions, herbal teas and gellulas are available to combat osteoporosis. A good remedy is a decoction of the aerial part of Horsetail. It is obtained by immersing 40 g of plant in a litre of water, and leaving to soak for around 8 hours. The mixture is boiled for a quarter of an hour and left to cool for 20 minutes. It is then mixed with another litre of water. The resulting solution should be taken in 3 cups a day for a month.

Sage tea is made by boiling a pinch of sage leaves in a cup of water for 3 minutes. The solution should be taken twice a day. Nettle is both remineralising and regenerating for the bone matrix, even consolidating fractures. Like Horsetail, it contains silica, but acts more on bone metabolism than on bone structure. A herbal tea is made by infusing 30 to 60 g of leaves per litre for 10 minutes in very hot, but not boiling, water. A 5-year study of 1,500 women suggests that regular consumption of tea helps to maintain good bone mineral density. It is important to note that Bamboo's high silica content means that it has the ability to maintain calcium metabolism and bone fixation by stimulating the synthesis of bone collagen. In addition, this trace element has a remineralising effect. It is therefore recommended for combating bone demineralisation (particularly in the spinal column). The shoots can be eaten and capsules purchased, while calcium is consumed at the same time. The capsules should be taken 3 times a day with a meal, if possible in combination with Alfa capsules. Bamboo capsules with cod liver oil help to strengthen bones and consolidate fractures. However, bamboo is not recommended for pregnant

[145] Sophie Laurent, "Les 10 oligo-éléments qui boostent la santé", *Femme Actuelle* 07/02 (2022) p.1-4.

women or children under the age of 7. Lithothame is a small seaweed that crystallises minerals, especially calcium carbonate. It helps maintain acid-base balance, as calcium carbonate is an anti-acid and is easily assimilated. It promotes bone remineralisation, ensuring bone growth and maintaining bone strength. Lithothame capsules should be taken 2 or 3 times a day with water, two per dose.

ovoid: Hybrid word formed from the Latin ovum (egg), and εἶδος, eidos (form). Word derived from ove, with the suffix -oid. Said of a leaf or fruit that has an oval shape, like that of an egg. An ovoid shape is a three-dimensional oval shape, or a shape reminiscent of an egg. In botany, an ovoid leaf or fruit has a globular, orbicular, oval or obovate shape. If there is little difference in diameter between the base and the apex, the shape is oblongoid.

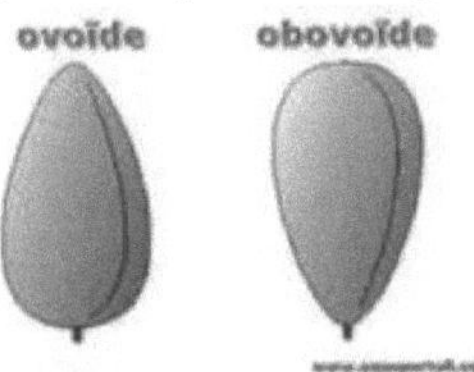

Comparison between ovoid and obovoid :

palmite: From the Spanish palmito (palmite). This is the edible pith of palm trees, which looks like curdled milk, is very tender and has a mild, pleasant flavour. It is also known as palm heart.

palmitine: Derived from palmite, with the suffix -ine. It is the triglyceride found in palm oil. Palmitin, discovered by Berthelot, can be prepared artificially with palmitic acid and glycerine. To extract it from palm oil, the oil is subjected to high pressure to remove the liquid fats, then the residue is boiled several times with 95 % alcohol. The free fatty acids dissolve in the alcohol, while the palmitin is insoluble.

palmitic: From palmitine, suff. -ic, from palmite. Palmitic acid is a fatty acid discovered by the French chemist Edmond Frémy in saponified palm oil. It is a saturated fatty acid, of animal origin or present in certain vegetable oils such as palm or coconut oil, but also in all oils and fats of vegetable or animal origin (meat, butter, milk, cheese). Example: candles made from palmitic acid and paraffin. Its chemical formula is $C_{16}H_{32}O_2$. They are called "omega-3" because their chemical structure has a common feature: it has an "unsaturation" on the third carbon. If we want to be more precise, omega-3s have several unsaturations (they are said to be polyunsaturated), the first of which is present on the third carbon. Omega-3 fatty acids are a family of essential fatty acids. They are essential fatty acids, necessary for the development and proper functioning of the human body, but which our body cannot produce.

panicle: From the Latin panicula, from panus (weaver's thread, thread in a bunch, spike with panicles). In botany, this is the compound inflorescence, a cluster of bunches. This is the inflorescence of certain grasses which takes the form of a cluster of spikelets whose more or less branched secondary axes decrease from the base to the top of the central axis. This is also known as a cluster arrangement. Example: flowers, fruit in panicles; millet bears its grains in panicles.

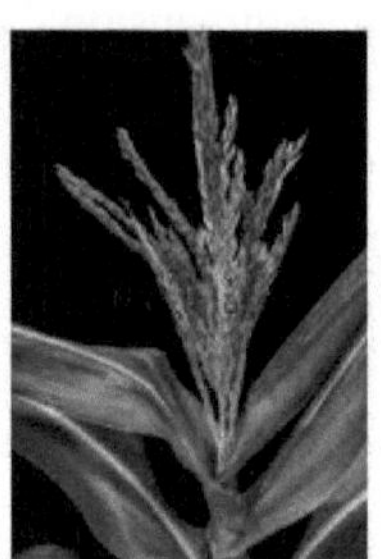
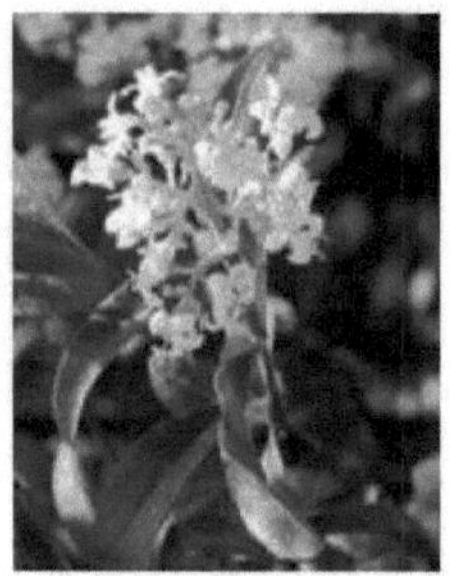
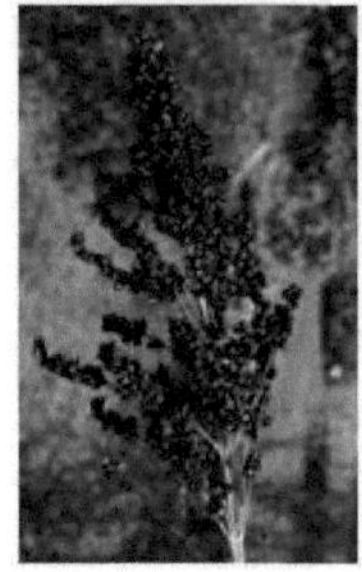

Panicle of corn Panicle of privet Panicle of Sorghum bicolor with ripening grins

pantothenic: from the Greek πάντοθεν, pántothen (everywhere). Refers to vitamin B $_5$, which is indeed found in almost all foods. It is found in particularly concentrated proportions in sprouts, wholemeal cereals and varieties of stinging nettle.

paralysis: From the ancient Greek παράλυσις, from παρά (indicating disturbance), and, λύσις, (dissolution). Paralysis or plegia is a loss of motor skills through reduction or loss of contractility of one or more muscles, due to damage to nerve pathways or muscles: if the phenomenon is incomplete, it is called paresis. Paralysis of nerve origin may be central or peripheral. Some metabolic diseases of the muscular system may cause paralysis without nerve or muscle damage (myasthenia). The degree of paralysis is graded from 0 to 5. At degree 0, there is no contraction (total paralysis or plegia), while at degree 1, there is visible contraction but no movement. Grade 2 is contraction allowing movement in the absence of gravity; grade 3 is contraction allowing movement against gravity; grade 4 is contraction allowing movement against resistance; finally grade 5 is normal muscle strength. A distinction is made between paralysis of central origin, due to a lesion in the brain, the brain stem or the spinal cord: paraplegia; quadriplegia (or tetraplegia); and paralysis of peripheral origin, due to damage to one or more roots, or one or more nerves, for example: radial paralysis; paralysis of the median nerve (as in carpal tunnel syndrome). Functional paralysis affects movements coordinated to carry out a specific type of action: for example, astasia-abasia (impaired walking and standing, but allowing other movements apart from walking).

Paraesthesia: From the ancient Greek παραίσθησις, paraísthesis: παρά, pará (beside, abnormal) and α'ίσθησις aísthêsis (sensation). It is a disorder of the sense of touch grouping several symptoms, the particularity of which is to be unpleasant but not painful: tingling, prickling, numbness. In medical terms, it is an unpleasant, non-painful sensitivity disorder that gives the sensation of feeling cotton wool, and can be accompanied by anaesthesia, tingling, skin stiffness and sometimes a "hot-cold" sensation.

pathology: in ancient Greek Παθολογία, pathologia, from πάθος, pathos (passion, disease) and λόγος logos (doctrine, study, science). It is the science whose object is the study of diseases, in particular their causes (aetiology) and mechanisms (physiopathology). It differs from nosology, which is concerned with the classification of diseases. Cardiac pathology is therefore the study of heart disease.

pedunculus: From the Latin pedunculus, diminutive of pes, pedis (foot). In botany, it is the stem or tail of a flower, after fertilisation, of a fruit, disticte of the stem of the plant. It is the axis bearing a flower or fruit. Its synonyms are: pedicel, tail, stem.

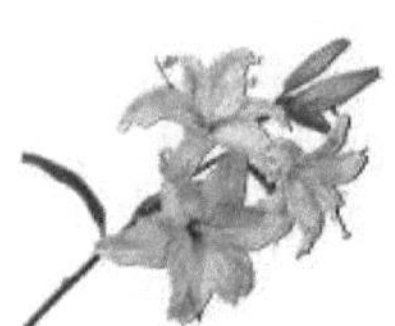
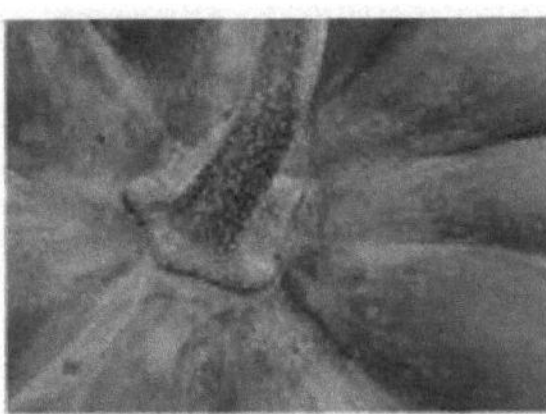

Lily stalk Squash stalk

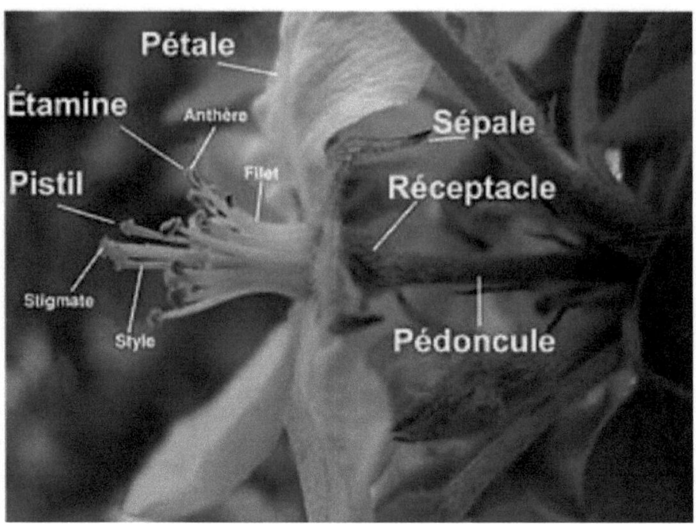

Apple blossom

phenol: From the ancient Greek φαίνω, phaino (to shine) and -ol. Phenol, also known as hydroxybenzene, phenic acid, or carbolic acid, is composed of a phenyl ring and a hydroxyl function. It is the simplest molecule in the phenol family. In organic chemistry, phenols are compounds consisting of an aromatic hydrocarbon ring (arene) and one or more hydroxyl groups -OH attached to it. Polyphenols, compounds made up of more than one phenolic ring, for example, are included among the phenols. Some phenols have important biological functions (biochemical defence against micro-organisms and fungi in plants in particular) in certain species, but they can be toxic to humans and other animal species. When they are abnormally disseminated in the environment, phenols are air, soil or water pollutants.

phlebitis: From the ancient Greek φλέψ, phleps (vein) with the medical suffix -ite, indicating inflammation. Phlebitis, or venous thrombosis, or thrombophlebitis is the formation of a blood clot (thrombus) in a vein, partially or completely blocking the passage of blood. In 90% of cases, it affects the calf and thigh. Superficial venous thrombosis is a complication of venous insufficiency. Deep phlebitis, on the other hand, is mainly the result of hypercoagulability. Symptoms include a feeling of heaviness in the leg, oedema in just one calf, hardening and swelling of the calf, sometimes extending as far as the thigh, and a bluish/purple discolouration of the affected area. Unlike simple varicose veins, phlebitis can have serious consequences when it is complicated by the migration of a blood clot into the pulmonary vessels.

porphyria: From the Greek πορφύρα, porphúra (purple). It is a hereditary disease caused by an abnormality in the synthesis of heme[146] , a pigment in haemoglobin, which leads to an accumulation of porphyrins in the tissues and exacerbated sensitivity to sunlight, causing skin lesions. It is also a group of rare diseases characterised by the accumulation of porphyrins in the body, affecting the skin and nervous system. Porphyrins are the main precursors of haem, an iron-containing pigment that is vital for all the body's organs. Acute porphyria induces intermittent attacks of abdominal, mental and neurological symptoms. These attacks are usually triggered by prescription drugs (including oral contraceptives), alcohol, smoking and other factors such as fasting, infections or stress. A different gene is altered for each type of acute porphyria. This mutation is inherited. As a result, a person with acute porphyria will often have family members who are "healthy" carriers of the same mutated gene. Cutaneous porphyria (CP) is the most common porphyria, affecting around one in every 25,000 of the population. In CP, porphyrins are produced in excess in the liver, accumulating throughout the body and causing the skin to become fragile and sensitive to light. Acute intermittent porphyria is due to a deficiency in the enzyme porphobilinogen deaminase (also known as hydroxymethylbilane synthase), which causes an accumulation of the porphyrin precursors delta-aminolevulinic acid and porphobilinogen, initially confined to the liver. Acute porphyrias are rare genetic disorders manifested by neurological and systemic symptoms, including abdominal pain, hyponatremia and seizures.

Hepatic porphyria manifests itself through the following symptoms: abdominal pain, sometimes acute or associated with lumbar pain radiating to the thighs; nausea, vomiting; constipation; confusion, convulsions, sensory loss and muscle weakness; psychiatric disorders (depression, mood disorders, anxiety, irritability), increased pulse rate and blood pressure; abnormal colouration of the urine; appearance of skin changes (sores then lesions). Attacks are often triggered by external risk factors: drugs contraindicated in the case of this disease (known as porphyrinogenic drugs); alcohol consumption; recurrent infections; low-calorie diet without medical supervision; stress, emotional shock.

In the event of an acute attack, the treatment involves an injection of human haemin and/or a carbohydrate infusion. This human haemin molecule regulates haem production by inhibiting the excessive production of an enzyme, thereby preventing the accumulation of neurotoxic precursors. Overall therapeutic management includes avoiding triggering factors, and protecting the skin from

---

[146] heme: a substance in the blood containing iron and porphyrin, whose role is to transport blood gases.

light to protect it from skin disorders[147] .
prophylaxis: From Ancient Greek προφυλακτικός, prophulaktikós (who protects, preserves; proctector), from προφύλαξη, prophylaxê (protection, prevention). It is the precaution proper to preserve from a disease. Prophylaxis, also known as prophylactic measures, refers to the active or passive process aimed at preventing the onset, spread or aggravation of a disease[148] , as opposed to curative therapy, which aims to cure it.
protein: From the ancient Greek πρωτεΐον, *prôteíon* (very first) with the suffix -ine. In a wide variety of forms, proteins play an essential role in the maintenance and renewal of tissues, and perform many functions at cell level: construction, functioning, defence. Proteins are chains of amino acids that can be found in muscles, skin, nails, hair, blood, many hormones, enzymes and antibodies, and are necessary for the growth, repair and defence of the body's tissues. They have a number of characteristics, including: macronutrients that are essential to life; amino acid compounds, both essential and non-essential, that define the quality of the protein; animal proteins and plant proteins are found in food; they play a wide range of roles in the body (enzymes, transport, tissue structure, etc.). In their energy role, they provide energy, i.e. 4 calories per gram. Like fats and carbohydrates, proteins are essential macronutrients for the body. C-reactive protein (or CRP) is a protein synthesised by the liver during inflammation. Measuring CRP is very common during a blood test, as it shows whether the body is coping with an attack. There are more than 20 natural amino acids in dietary proteins, nine of which are important amino acids that the body cannot manufacture. They must therefore be obtained through the diet. The other amino acids are non-essential because the body can produce them. Some proteins are digestive enzymes that enable food molecules to be assimilated, while others form antibodies and enable the body to defend itself against external aggression. They also form the basis of haemoglobin and certain hormones.
Proteins form a large family: *amino acids*, peptides and *proteins*. They are also called *nitrogen compounds* because they all contain nitrogen. The food with the highest protein content is spirulina, which provides 57.5g of protein per 100g of 30 foods. For example, dry salted cod: 47.6 g, grison meat: 38.9 g. Because of

[147] "Acute hepatic porphyria: symptoms and treatment of this rare disease", Passeport Santé, consulted on 29/07/2023 (https://www.passeportsante.net/fr/Maux/Problemes/Fiche.aspx?doc=acute-hepatic-porphyria-symptoms-treatment-this-rare-disease) p. 1-4.
[148] Centre National de Ressources Textuelles et Lexicales (CNRTL), "Definition of prophylaxis", Co-consulted on 30/06/ 2023 (https://www.cnrtl.fr/definition/academie9/prophylaxie).

their origin, there are two types of protein: animal and vegetable. In chemistry, the term protide is used to refer to amino acids and all their derivatives: oligopeptides, polypeptides, proteins, etc. Proteins are often mistakenly referred to as "proteins". In reality, proteins are a large family grouping together several molecules, including proteins. DNA is located in the nucleus of the cell, while protein synthesis takes place in the cytoplasm. There is an intermediary capable of moving from the nucleus to the cytoplasm to transport the genetic information to the protein synthesis machinery. This intermediary is called messenger RNA. We recommend eating animal proteins every day: meat, fish and eggs, with a high protein intake. Proteins are complete because they provide all the essential amino acids, like eggs.

pyrexia: from the ancient Greek πυρεσσειν, puressein (to have a fever), from πυρ, pyr (fire, fever). It is a feverish state and conversely, apyrexia is synonymous with the absence of fever. Fever is defined as a rise in body temperature above 38°C. Between 37.7°C and 37.9°C, it is called febrile. The temperature can be taken in the rectum, the most reliable measurement, but also in the armpit (add 0.5°C) and in the mouth (add 0.4°C). A distinction should be made between fever and lihyperthermia, both of which cause an increase in body temperature, but result from different mechanisms. Fever is a pathological phenomenon triggered in certain contexts by substances called pyrogens[149] .

root: From the Low Latin radĭcĭna, a diminutive of the Latin radix (root, base, source, foundation) from which comes the Old French rais (root) which gives horseradish and radish. It is generally the underground organ of vascular plants, which attaches them to the soil and provides them with water and mineral salts. There are four types of root: stilt roots, which support the trunk above the ground or water (mangrove); aerial roots (epiphytic orchids); liana roots (banyan); sucker roots (vanilla).

Rhinopharyngitis (or nasopharyngitis, commonly known as the common cold) is a frequent and generally benign infection of the upper airways (nasal cavity and pharynx) by a virus, mainly picornaviridae (including rhinoviruses), adenoviruses or coronaviruses. The main symptoms of the common cold are rhinitis (sneezing, congestion and nasal discharge of mucus), an infrequent and delayed dry or productive cough, pharyngitis, conjunctivitis, phlegm, fatigue, headaches, but generally no fever (if there is one, especially in children where it is common, it does not exceed 38.5 - 39°C), loss of appetite and diffuse pain (in

---

149 "Pyrexia and apyrexia", Ooreka Santé, Accessed 18/06/2023 (https://premiers- secours.ooreka.fr/astuce/voir/724289/pyrexie-et-apyrexie) 1-2.

half the cases). It is the most common respiratory infection in young children.
Rheumatology: From the ancient Greek ρεῦμα, rheûma then from the Latin rheuma (flow, flowing), and from λόγος logos (doctrine, study, science). It is a medical speciality concerned with the diagnosis and treatment of diseases of the musculoskeletal system, i.e. diseases of the bones, joints, muscles, tendons and ligaments. The diseases can be divided into the following groups: osteoarthritis, osteoporosis, gout, low back pain, rheumatoid arthritis and spondyloarthritis.
Rheumatologist: From the ancient Greek ρεῦμα, rheûma then from the Latin rheuma (flow, flowing). and from λόγος logos (doctrine, study, science). It is the doctor specializing in rheumatology, also treat certain peripheral neurological conditions such as sciatica and especially all inflammatory rheumatism and autoimmune diseases that can have many extra-articular manifestations: skin, eyes, kidneys, lungs.
cold: From the Low Latin rheuma (flowing water, marine flux, or catarrh). The term itself is borrowed from the Greek ρεῦμα (fluxion), from ρεἰν (to flow). In addition to rhinopharyngitis, the term can also refer to rhinitis caused by hay fever (allergic rhinitis), pollen allergy, the common cold (coryza) and other types of infection such as synovitis (hip colds).
sclerosis: From the ancient Greek σκλήρωσις, sclerosis (hardening). It is the pathological hardening of an organ or tissue or lesion caused by excessive collagen formation (abnormal development of fibrous connective elements) or, in the case of the nervous system, demyelination. This is an elementary lesion in dermatological pathology. It may involve abnormal stiffening of the skin. It may be localised or generalized to the entire cutaneous integument. Sclerosis is often secondary to mechanical, chemical or physical processes. The primitive nature of skin sclerosis is observed in scleroderma. Sclerosis is also a treatment technique used in phlebology, where a sclerosing product is injected into varicosities or varicose veins to neutralise them.
scurvy: this is a disease caused by a deficiency in vitamin C (ascorbic acid) which, in the most serious forms, leads to loosening of the teeth, purulent gums, haemorrhaging and, finally, death.
Scorpioid: From the Greek Skorpion, scorpion (scorpion) and eidh, eidè (form, appearance). In botany, this refers to a leguminous plant with a spiky, rolled-up pod that bears some resemblance to a scorpion's tail. Also used to describe a plant used to make a remedy for scorpion stings.

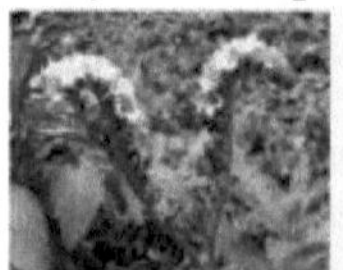
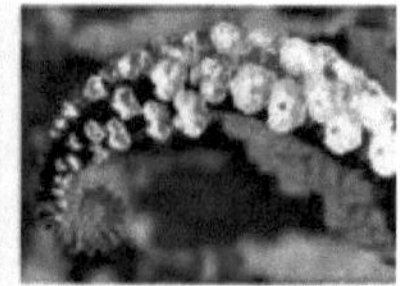

The scorpioid inflorescence of Heliotropium indicum

And a scorpioid organ has a rolled shape like a scorpion's tail or a crozier. Scorpioid refers to a uniparous cyme in which a single bud takes over the growth of the axis and always on the same side, causing the cyme to roll up like a scorpion's tail. The tip of a fern branch is often scorpioid. A scorpioid cyme is one in which the axis is curved and the flowers appear in two rows and on alternate sides of the axis (as with forget-me-nots). It can be : a one-sided cymose inflorescence, curled to resemble a scorpion's tail; a two-sided cymose inflorescence, curled to resemble a scorpion's tail, with single flowers alternating on the right and left; a zigzag inflorescence with branches developing alternately on opposite sides of the rachis; circinate at the tip (like unilateral racemes); cymose and unilateral, coiled to resemble the tail of a scorpion, as in the Boraginaceae.

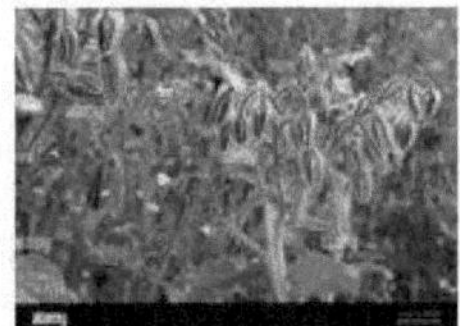
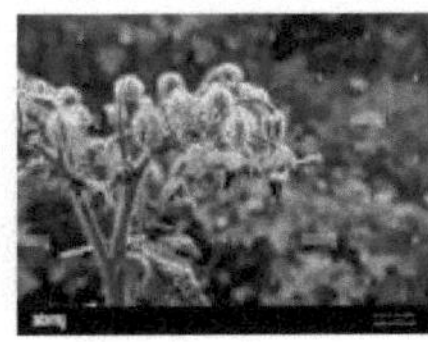
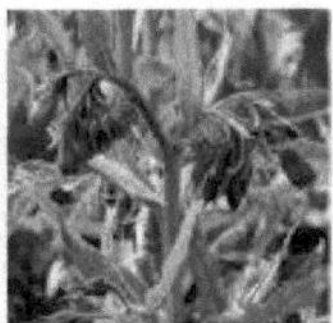

Form of scorpioid cyme.

sepal: From Latin sepalum, from Ancient Greek σκέπη, skepê (cover) with the Greek final πέταλον, petalon (leaf). In botany, this refers to each of the parts forming the calyx (outer whorl) of a flower. It is each of the foliate elements, usually green, whose union composes the calyx and supports the corolla of the flower. The calyx may be synadelphous or idiadelphous (monosepal or polysepal) and each of these divisions, taken separately, is called a sepal. Sepals may be toothed, erect, free or fused. This name is more generally used for the divisions of the idiadelph calyx; those of the synadelph calyx, called teeth or lobes by botanists, are nonetheless sepals that have been fused over part of their length. The flower of the jatropha, for example, is an actinomorph, unisexual with a calyx of 5 sepals and a corolla of 5 free petals.

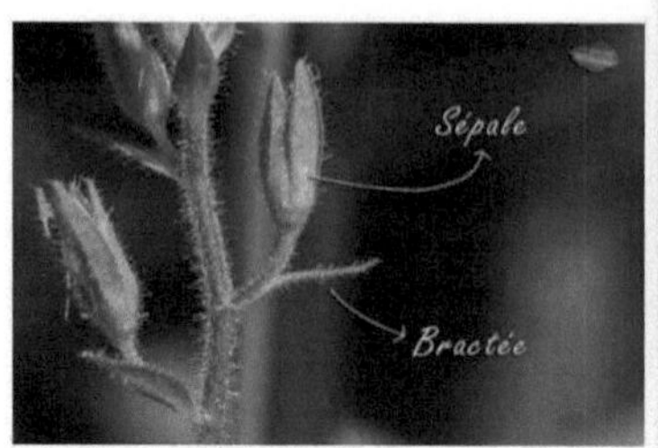

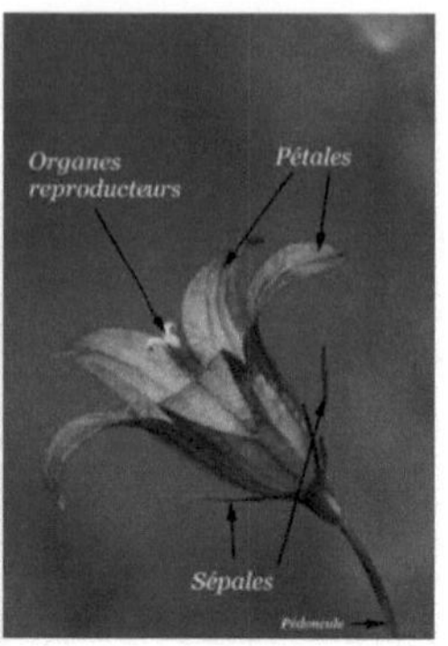

sialagogue: From the ancient Greek σίαλον, sialon (saliva) and αγωγός agôgos from αγειν, agein, (which brings, which leads). In pharmacology, it refers to the drug that stimulates salivary secretion.

spasm: From Latin spasmus, from Greek σπασμός, from σπάω (to pull, to contract). Pathological contraction of muscles and especially smooth muscles. The most frequent spasms are those in the hollow organs and sphincters: digestive tract, urinary tract and respiratory system.) *spasmodic*: from Latin spasmus, from Greek σπασμός, spasmos from σπάω, spao (to pull, contract). Which is of the nature of spasm; which is caused, marked, affected by spasms, muscular contractions.

squamiform: From the Latin squama (scale), with the suffix -form. In botany, this refers to the semi-amplexicaul, short, broad, scale-like leaves of the nectaries, which have the shape of one of the squamellae, no different from the squames or bracts of the pericline.

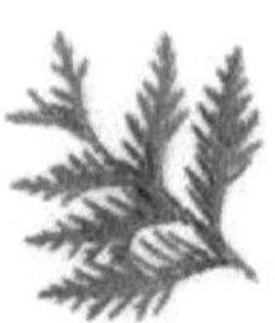

squamiform leaf (or scale)

Steroid: from the Greek στερεός, stereós (solid, firm, hard, resistant, cruel, harsh, difficult). It is a generic name for hormones derived from sterols, secreted by the endocrine glands (adrenocortical glands, genital glands [testes and ovaries], placenta). It is also a body derived from sterols, non-saponifiable, insoluble in water and soluble in organic solvents, characterised by a tetracyclic nucleus. In biochemistry, it is a lipid derived from triterpenoids (lipids with 30 carbon atoms), mainly squalene, and is characterised by a nucleus with four hydrophobic cyclopentanophenanthrenic carbon rings derived from a sterane, cholesterol, partially or totally hydrogenated. There are a large number of anabolic steroids used illegally, of which the most commonly used today are testosterone, Stanozolol, Metandienone, Nandrolone and Oxandrolol - the substances are injected or taken orally. Anabolic steroids are mainly used to promote growth in farm animals. They are sometimes prescribed to humans to treat delayed puberty, certain types of impotence and weight loss due to AIDS and other *sterol* diseases. In biochemistry, sterol is the complex polycyclic alcohol found in animals, plants and fungi. It is a lipid with a sterane ring whose carbon 3 carries a hydroxyl group. Sterols are considered a subclass of steroids. Cholesterol (in all eukaryotes) and polysterols (mainly in plants) are sterols present in cell membranes and play a central role in many biochemical processes. In animals, cholesterol is vital for cell function, and is a precursor of fat-soluble vitamins and steroid hormones. Sterols are present in small quantities in certain plants (cereals, vegetable oils, vegetables, fruit, nuts, etc.) and are therefore naturally supplied by the usual diet, but in very small quantities (400 mg/day on average).

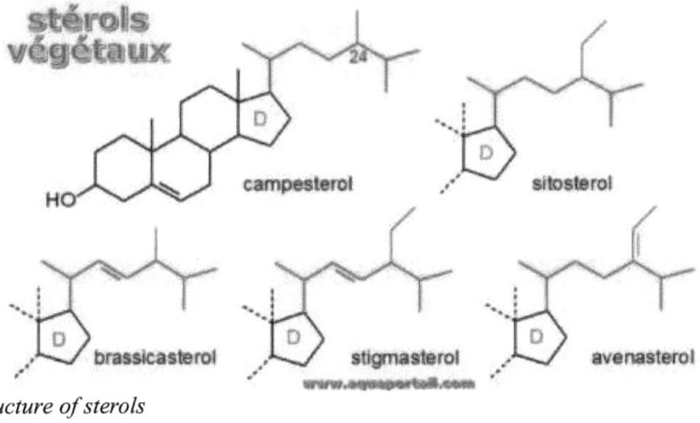

Molecular structure of sterols

With a biochemical structure very similar to that of cholesterol, plant sterols play a role similar to that of cholesterol in humans in maintaining the structural and functional integrity of cell membranes. In humans, intestinal absorption of plant sterols is low. Plant sterols bind to the micelles that transport cholesterol in the intestine, reducing its absorption through competition. Unabsorbed cholesterol is then eliminated in the faeces, leading to a reduction in LDL[150] - cholesterol (known as 'bad' cholesterol) in the blood.

[150] *Low-density lipoproteins* are a group of lipoproteins of varying types and sizes (18 to 25 nm in diameter). Their function is to transport cholesterol, free or esterified, in the blood and throughout the body to the cells. LDL is produced by the liver from *low-density lipoprotein* (*VLDL*). They contain apolipoprotein *B-100*, a monolayer of phospholipids, triglycerides and fat-soluble antioxidant vitamins (vitamin E and carotenoids).

stomachic: In ancient Greek στομαχικός, stomakhikós (of the stomach, good for the stomach), derived from στόμαχος, stómakhos (oesophagus). It refers to that which is beneficial to the stomach, which aids digestion.
symptom: In ancient Greek σύμπτωμα, accident; from σύν, syn- (with), and πίπτειν, piptein (to fall).The word σύμπτωμα / símptoma, in Greek, means encounter, coincidence; it is derived from the verb συμπίπτω / sumpíptõ (to occur at the same time, to meet, to coincide), with the suffix -μα / -ma. A symptom is originally "that which occurs together", that which "co-incides", in the literal sense of the word. In medicine, a symptom or functional sign is a sign that represents a manifestation of a disease, as observed in a patient. They are clinical warning signs that the patient complains of (such as pain, cough, dizziness or sadness). We can distinguish: physical signs, discovered by examining the patient: abdominal contracture, murmur; certain general signs: fever, high blood pressure; paraclinical signs obtained with the help of complementary examinations: radiological signs following X-rays, biological signs following samples.
terpenes: From the German Terpen from das Terpentin (the terebinthine). Terpenes are a class of hydrocarbons produced by many plants, particularly conifers. They are major components of resin and of the terebinthin essence produced from resin. Terpenes are secondary metabolites that are also found in metazoans (pheromones and sesquiterpene hormones in hexapods, diterpenes in aquatic organisms (cnidarians, sponges).
tonic: In ancient Greek τονικός, tonikós (tone, tonus). It refers to that which has an elastic tension, speaking of tissues, muscles, that which offers renitence and elasticity, which fortifies, stimulates the organism: a fortifier, a stimulant, a tonic. In pathology, we speak of tonic spasms when we are talking about regular contractions that are still subject to the will, as opposed to clonic spasms. Medicines which have the ability to slowly and insensibly stimulate the organic action of the various systems of the animal economy, and to increase their strength in a lasting way, are also called tonics. Cinchona, for example, is a tonic.
terpenoid: From the German Terpen (from "das Terpentin", turpentine) and the Greek terpen, terpen and eidoV, eidos (aspect, form). It is a naturally occurring organic molecule belonging to the terpene family. These compounds are derived from isoprene, an unsaturated hydrocarbon. They are characterised by their cyclic structure and chemical diversity. They are responsible for the aromas and flavours of many plants such as fruit, flowers and spices. Some have anti-inflammatory, antimicrobial or antioxidant properties. Terpenes are basic hydrocarbons, while terpenoids contain additional functional groups. These

lipids can be found in all classes of living creatures, and constitute the largest group of natural products. They contribute to the fragrance of eucalyptus, the taste of cinnamon, cloves and ginger and the yellow colours of flowers. Known terpenoids include citral, menthol, camphor and cannabinoids found in the Cannabis plant. Terpenoids can be thought of as modified terpenes, with methyl groups added or removed, or oxygen atoms added (some authors use the term 'terpene' more broadly, including terpenoids). Like terpenes, terpenoids can be classified according to their number of isoprenic units and their number of C5n carbon atoms: hemiterpenoids, 1 isoprenic unit, in C5; monoterpenoids, 2 isoprenic units, in C10; sesquiterpenoids, 3 isoprenic units, in C15; diterpenoids, 4 isoprenic units, in C20 ; sesterterpenoids, 5 isoprenic units, in C25; triterpenoids, 6 isoprenic units, in C30; tetraterpenoids, 8 isoprenic units, in C40; polyterpenoids with a larger number of isoprenic units.

Therapeutik: From Ancient Greek θεραπευτικός, therapeutikós (attentive, helpful, curative, maintenance, treatment, care of the body, medical care, treatments, preparation of a remedy). From qerapeuin therapeuein (to heal). Medicine is the study and teaching of how to treat illnesses and how to cure and relieve the sick. It is also the set of methods used to combat disease and to restore and preserve health. Its synonym is therapy.

therophyte: From the ancient Greek θέρος, theros (summer; good season) and φυτόν, phutón (plant). These are plants with an annual cycle that survive the bad season in the form of seeds, all vegetative parts being destroyed by desiccation due to frost or drought. They are summer or winter annuals and develop rapidly.

thrombosis: Greek θρομβός, thrombós (rounded grain, clot), and the suffix -ose disease. It is the abnormal formation of a blood clot in the lumen of an arterial vessel (example: coronary thrombosis), venous vessel (example: thrombophlebitis of the lower limbs) or in a cavity of the heart with a local inflammatory and painful reaction. Venous thrombosis can be superficial, when it affects the small veins located between the skin and the muscles, or deep when it involves a larger vein. The term "cerebral thrombosis" refers to an obstruction caused by a blood clot that has migrated into a cerebral artery, leading to ischaemia of the downstream tissue and a stroke.

stem: From the Latin tibia (flute, main leg bone). In botany, it is the part of a plant that emerges from the earth and from which branches, leaves, flowers and fruit grow. An axis-shaped plant organ that connects its basic organs: leaves and roots. There are three types of stem: aerial stems, underground stems and aquatic stems.

tisane: From lat. ptisana, tisana (hulled barley; barley decoction), from ancient Greek πτισάνη, ptisáne (oat brouet), barley decoction being, in ancient medicine, one of the main remedies against fever and serving as a base for infusions or decoctions of plants. This is a drink obtained by macerating, infusing or decocting plants in water, often with medicinal properties. Examples: barley tea, cherry stem tea, neem tea, quinqueliba tea; soothing, calming, depurative, diuretic, emollient, purgative, refreshing, sudorific teas; lemon tea.

trypanocide: From ancient Greek τρύπανον trúpanon (instrument for piercing, auger, trepan), Latin cædere (to strike, beat, break, split, slaughter, kill, massacre). Used to describe a drug active against trypanosomiasis. In African trypanosomiasis, sodium suramin or pentamidine are used parenterally in the lymphatico-sanguine phase; melarsoprol containing trivalent arsenic, especially in the meningoencephalitis phase; and difluoromethylornithine (DFMO), an ornithine decarboxylase inhibitor, can be combined with nifurtimox. In South American trypanosomiasis, two derivatives of nitroheterocycles are used: niflurtimox and benznidazole, administered buccally and active only during the acute phase.

Varicose vein: This is the permanent dilation of a vein, produced by the accumulation of blood in its cavity, most often on a lower limb. Varicose veins of the lower limbs are dilated subcutaneous veins with a diameter greater than 3 mm. Varicose veins are usually sinuous. They are the site of blood reflux.

vermifuge: From the Latin vermis (worm) and -fuge, fugare (to chase away). A medicine that destroys or expels intestinal worms. Synon.

xanthone: From the ancient Greek ξανθός, *xanthós* (yellow), as these molecules are yellow in colour. In chemistry, this word in the singular refers to a substance with the gross formula $C_{13}H_8O_2$, it is the leader of many other molecules found in various plants: xanthones in the plural, or xantanoids. Xanthone is also a **name for dibenzo-γ-pyrone and, by extension, all compounds with this skeleton. Natural xanthones are plant polyphenolic pigments of**
yellow in colour, existing in the free state or in the form of heterosides (*O*- and *C*-*heterosides*). They are found in particular in *Gentianaceae* (e.g. gentian) and *Clusiaceae* (e.g. mangosteen, *Garcinia mangostana* L., whose fruit, mangosteen, contains many xanthones).

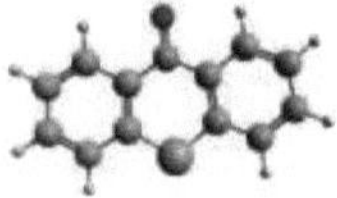

Xanthone molecule

Xanthonoids or xanthones are a class of natural phenols whose structure is derived from xanthone. They are natural yellow pigments present in many plants, particularly flowers. They are found in particular in members of the

Clusiaceae family. Some xanthonoids are thought to have anti-inflammatory, antispasmodic, antidiuretic and antiseptic properties. Examples include : tomentonone, zeyloxanthonone and calozeyxanthonone isolated from the bark of *Calophyllum tomentosum,* a flowering plant from Sri Lanka; apetalinones A, B, C and D found in *Calophyllum apetalum*; gaudichaudiones A, B, C, D, E, F, G and H, gaudichaudiic acids A, B, C, D and E, morellic acid and forbesione in *Garcinia morella*; methhylswertianine and bellidifoline in Swertia punicea; psorospermine in *Psorospermum febrifugum*; cassiaxanthone in *Cassia reticulata*. It is important to highlight the existence of cytotoxic xanthones (gamogin, morelline, dimethylacetal, isomreollin B, moréollic acid, gambogenic acid, gambogenin, isogambogenin, deoxygambogenin, gambogenin dimethylacetal, gambogellic acid, isomerelline, morellic acid, deoxymorelline and nanburin) which have been isolated from *Garcinia hanburyi* latex. Xanthones have antioxidant, anti-cancer, anti-inflammatory, anti-allergic and anti-microbial (bacteria, fungi and viruses) properties.

xerophile: From the ancient Greek ξερος, xeros (dry) and φιλος, philos: friend). Refers to extremophilic organisms living in environments that are very poor in water. They include bacteria, fungi, plants (sometimes called xerophytes), insects, nematodes and the shrimp Artemia salina, which can tolerate extreme desiccation. Teminology is especially used for plants in extremely dry environments, in very poor soils, formed in superficial layers, or in soils that are dry either due to a lack of substrate or due to the climate. Xerophilous plants include: aloe, agave, opuncias, candle cactus, mother-in-law's cushion, witch's claw, lithops, as well as caudex plants, baobab and yucca.

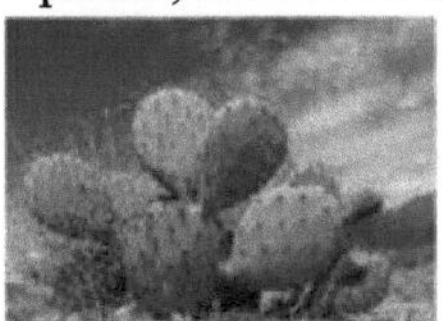

Gamm vert

CONCLUSION

The *baobab* in Fon *Kpassa*, the unscientific *Adansonia digitata*, is found in Africa, Madagascar, the Indian Ocean islands, Australia and the Caribbean. The trunk, with its spongy tissues, can store up to 100,000 litres of water for sedentary communities and nomadic tribes. It is rich in proteins, lipids, carbohydrates, mucilage, vitamins A, B1, B2, B6 and C, essential amino acids and minerals including sodium (Na), magnesium (Mg), calcium (Ca), potassium (K) and iron (Fe). It also contains flavonoids and phenolic acids. It is an antioxidant and inhibitor of enzymatic activity, anti-carcinogenic, antimicrobial and anti-inflammatory, antisickling, antibacterial, antidiabetic, antirheumatic, antitrypanosome, arthritic, antioxidant, antiviral, analgesic, antipyretic, diuretic and hepatoprotective, tonic/stimulant, antidiarrhoeal, antienteralgic, antipyretic, Its extracts are effective against fatigue, inappetence, diarrhoea, enteralgia, nasopharyngeal infections, circulatory disorders (haemorrhoids), haemoptysis, insect bites and dermatitis. It plays a symbolic and ritual role in the mystique of health and the quest for fertility.

The pulp is used in various preparations for its binding, thickening and acidifying properties, in the composition of numerous cereal preparations such as porridges or couscous (for example, "mutchoyan" in Benin or "ngalakh" in Senegal), sauces or accompanying creams (for example, sweet cream made from roasted and crushed groundnuts in Senegal). It is sometimes used to coagulate milk, to activate the alcoholic fermentation of drinks made from sugarcane juice or cereal beers, or to thicken cooked sweet preparations made from local fruit (mango, orange, ditax, etc.). It is added to milk to make sweet drinks rich in vitamin C or sorbets. The seed powder can be used as a coffee substitute. Seed oil has a special place in cooking. When crushed, the seeds are used as a thickener in many sauces and soups, or in combination with other ingredients such as peanuts and sesame seeds. They are also used to make sweet creams. The young leaves are eaten raw or boiled as vegetables in sauces to accompany couscous, rice or other cereal-based dishes such as millet, sorghum or maize. The powdered dried leaves are used as a binding agent in the preparation of millet couscous.

BIBLIOGRAPHY

6.1 Monographs

Assogbadjo A.E., *Importance socio-économique et étude de la variabilité écologique, morphologique, génétique et biochimique du baobab (Adansonia digitata L.) au Bénin.* PhD thesis. Faculty of Bioscience Engineering, Ghent University, Belgium (2006) 213 p.

Boullard Bernard , *Plantes & Champignons*, Éditions Estem, 1997, 878 p.

Codjia T. C. et als, *Le baobab, une espèce à usage multiple au Bénin.* Cotonou, Benin, 2001.

Colasanti J. et al, *The maize floral transition. Bennetzen JL*, (2009) (eds) Handbook of Maize: Its Biology, Springer, New York, USA, p 41-55.

Diop Aidda Gabar, *The African baobab (Adansonia digitata L.): main characteristics and uses* Cambridge University Press, (2006).

Hitchcock, A. S.. 1971, *Manual of the grasses of the United States. Courier Corporation, US Department of Agriculture* (1971).

Norman M. J. T. et als, *The ecology of tropical food crops*. Cambridge University Press (1995).

Norman M. J. T. et als, *The ecology of tropical food crops*. Cambridge University Press (1995).

Ogbaga C. C. et als, *Phytochemical, Elemental and Proximate Analyses of Stored, Sun-Dried and Shade-Dried Baobab (Adansonia Digitata*) Leaves. 2017
.

Sidibe M. et als, *Adansonia Digitata L. Fruits for the future 4. International Center for Underutilized Crops (ICUC): University of Southampton, Southampton*, UK 2002.

Sidibe M. et als, *Baobab, Adansonia Digitata L. Fruits for the future 4. International Center for Underutilized Crops (ICUC)*: University of Southampton, Southampton, UK 2002.

Wickens G. A , *The Uses of the Baobab (Adansonia digitata L.) in Africa. In: Browse in Africa*. ILRI (aka ILCA and ILRAD): Addis-Ababa, Ethiopia 1980.

6.2 Articles

Abiona D. et als, "Proximate Analysis, Phytochemical Screening and Antimicrobial Activity of Baobab (Adansonia digitata) Leaves", . *IOSR JAC 8 (*2015) p. 60-65.

Abioye V. F.et als, "Effects of different drying methods on the nutritional and quality attributes of baobab leaves (Adansonia digitata)", *Agric. Biol. J. N. Am 5 (*2014) p. 104-108.

Adanson M., "Description d'un arbre nouveau genre appelé Baobab, observé au Sénégal", *Hist. Acad. Roy. Sci.* (Paris) (1791) p. 218-243.

Adida Sarah , "Fever: what is it? Passeport Santé 28/12 (2022) 1-2.
Al-Qarawi A. A. et als, "Hepatoprotective Influence of Adansonia digitata Pulp", *Journal of Herbs, Spices & Medicinal Plants* 10 (2003) p. 1-6.
Aluko A. E., et als, "Nutritional Quality and Functional Properties of Baobab (Adansonia digitata) Pulp from Tanzania", *Journal of Food Research* 5/23 (2016).
Anne-Sohie O. 10 aliments anti-cancer à privilégier", Radis 06/09 (2021) 1-2.
Assogbadjo A.E. et als, "Caractères morphologiques et production des capsules de baobab (Adansonia digitata L.) au Bénin", *Fruits* 60/5 (2005) p. 327-340.
Assogbadjo A.E. et als, "Ecological diversity and pulp, seed and kernel production of the baobab (Adansonia digitata) in Benin", *Belgian Journal of Botany* 138/1 (2005) p. 47-56.
Assogbadjo A.E. et als, "Genetic fingerprinting using AFLP cannot distinguish traditionally classified baobab morphotypes", *Agroforestry Systems* 75 (2009) p. 157-165.
Assogbadjo A.E. et al, "Caractérisation et stratégies de conservation du baobab (Adansonia digitata L.) dans les paysages agraires du Bénin", . In: Mayaka T.B., De longh H. and Sinsin B. (eds) (2007). *Ecological restoration of African Savanna Ecosystems. Proceedings of the third RNSCC International Seminar, 6 Feb, Cotonou, Benin. CEDC/CML*, Leiden University (2007) p. 35-50.
Assogbadjo A. E. als, "Caractères morphologiques et production des capsules de baobab (Adansonia digitata L.) au Bénin", *Fruits* 60/5 /09 (2005) p. 327-340.
Assogbadjo A.E. et als, "Folk classification, perception and preferences of baobab products in West Africa: consequences for species conservation and improvement", *Economic Botany* 62/1 (2008) p. 74-84.
Assogbadjo A.E. et als, "Patterns of genetic and morphometric diversity in baobab (Adansonia digitata L.) populations across different climatic zones of Benin (West Africa)", *Annals of botany* 97 2006) p. 819-830.
Assogbadjo A. E. et als, "Variation in biochemical composition of baobab (Adansonia digitata) pulp, leaves and seeds in relation to soil types and tree provenances", *Agriculture, Ecosystems & Environment* 157 (2012) p. 157, 94-99.
Aylor D. E., "Rate of dehydration of corn (*Zea mays*) pollen in the air". *Journal of Experimental Biology* 54/391 (2003) p. 2307-2312.
Baidoo I. K. et als, "Major, Minor and Trace Element Analysis of Baobab Fruit and Seed by Instrumental Neutron Activation Analysis Technique", *Food and Nutrition Sciences* 04 (2013) pp. 772-778.
Bannert M. et al, "Cross-pollination of maize at long distance", *European Journal of Agronomy* 27/1 (2007) p. 44-51.

Barker D. H. et als, "Internal and external photoprotection in developing leaves of the CAM plant Cotyledon orbiculata", Plant, Cell & Environnement, vol. 20 5 (1997) p. 617-624 (DOI 10.1111/j.1365-3040.1997.00078.x).
Baum, D. A. et al, "A review of chromosome numbers in Bombacaceae with new counts for Adansonia", *Taxon* 43/1 (1994) p. 11-20.
Baum D. A., "A systematic revision of Adansonia, Bombacaceae", *Annals of the Missouri Botanical Garden 82* (1995) p. 440-470.
Bolaños J. et al, "The importance of the anthesis-silking interval in breeding for drought tolerance in tropical maize", *Field Crops Research* 48 (1996) p. 65-.
Bonhomme R.M.et als, "Flowering of diverse maize cultivars in relation to temperature and photoperiod in multilocation field trials", *Crop Science* 34 (1994) p. 156-164.
Caron Michel "Glycine: what is it?", Futura 02/05 (2023) p. 1-3.
Chadare F. J. et als, "Baobab Food Products: A Review on their Composition and Nutritional Value", *Critical Reviews in Food Science and Nutrition* 49 (2009) p. 254-274.
Chadare F. J. et als, (2008), "Indigenous Knowledge and Processing of Adansonia Digitata L. Food Products In Benin", *Ecology of Food and Nutrition* 47 (2008) p. 47: 1-25.
Cisse M. et als, "Caractérisation du fruit du baobab et étude de sa transformation en nectar", *Fruits 64 (*2009) p. 64, 19-34.
Codjia, J.T.C. et als, 001). "Le baobab (Adansonia digitata), une espèce à usage multiple au Bénin. *Coco Multimédia, Cotonou, Benin* (2001).
Coe E. H. et als, "The genetics of corn." (1988) p. 81-257 *in* F. Sprague, J. W. Dudley, eds. Corn and Corn Improvement (Third Edition), Madison, Wisconsin, USA.
Cook B. G. et als, "Tropical Forages: an interactive selection tool", Accessed on 24/08/2023 (https://www.tropicalforages.info/text/intro/index.html) p. 1.
De Caluwé E. et als, (2008). "Ethnic differences in use value and use patterns of baobab (Adansonia digitata L.) in northern Benin", *African Journal of Ecology* (2008).
Diop Aïda Gabar et als, "Le baobab africain (Adansonia digitata L.) : principales caractéristiques et utilisations", *Fruits* 61/1 (2005) p.
55-69.
Douie C. et als, "Verifying the presence of the newly discovered African baobab, Adansonia kilima, in Zimbabwe through morphological analysis", *South African Journal of Botany* 100 (2015) pp. 164-168.
Edogbanya O. P. Comparative Study of the Proximate Composition of Edible Parts of Adansonia digitata L. obtained from Zaria, Kaduna State, Nigeria.

MAYFEB", *Journal of Biology and Medicine* 1 (2016).
Florimond A., Pothet A., "Méristème végétatif" on ens-lyon.fr (consulted on 28/06/ 2023).
Gaiwe R. et als, "Calcium and mucilage in the leaves of Adansonia digitata (Baobab)", *International Journal of Crude Drug Research 27 (*1989,) p. 101-104.
Ghedira K., "Flavonoids: structure, biological properties, prophylactic role and therapeutic uses", Phytotherapie, vol. 3 4 (2005) p. 162 (DOI 10.1007/s10298-005-0096-8).
Gordon C. M.et als, "Functional hypothalamic amenorrhea: An Endocrine Society Clinical Practice Guideline". J Clin Endocrinol Metab 102 /5 (2017) p. 1413-1439, 2017.
Hall A. J. et als, "Water stress before and during flowering in maize and its effects on yield, its components, and their determinants", *Maydica* 26 (1981) p. 26:19-38.
Hyacinthe T. et als, "Variability of vitamins B1, B2 and minerals content in baobab (Adansonia digitata) leaves in East and West Africa", *Food Science & Nutrition* 3 (2015) p. 3, 17-24.
Jensen J. S. et als, "A research approach supporting domestication of Baobab (Adansonia digitata L.) in West Africa", *New Forests* 41 (2011) p. 317-335.
Kerharo J et al, La pharmacopée sénégalaise traditionnelle - Plantes médicinales et toxiques, Vigot Frères, Paris, France, 1974.
Kamatou G. P. P. et als, "An updated review of Adansonia digitata: A commercially important African tree", *South African Journal of Botany* 77 (2011) pp. 908-919.
Kerharo J., "Le baobab, (Adansonia digitata), panacée africaine", *Quarterly Journal of Crude Drug Research:* 9/3 (1969) p. 1401-1408. Online publication 27/09 (2008).
Khakimov B. et als, "A comprehensive and comparative GC-MS metabolomics study of non-volatiles in Tanzanian grown mango, pineapple, jackfruit, baobab and tamarind fruits",. *Food Chemistry* 213 (2016) p. 691-699.
Osman M. A., "Chemical and nutrient analysis of baobab (Adansonia digitata) fruit and seed protein solubility", *Plant Foods for Human Nutrition (Formerly Qualitas Plantarum) 59 (*2004) p. 29-33.
Kim E. O. et als, "Anti-inflammatory activity of hydroxycinnamic acid derivatives isolated from corn bran in lipopolysaccharide-stimulated Raw 264.7 macrophages", *Food and Chemical Toxicology* 50 (2012) pp. 1309-1316.
Kyndt T. et als, "Spatial genetic structuring of baobab (Adansonia digitata, Malvaceae) in the traditional agroforestry systems of West Africa", *American*

Journal of Botany 96 (2009) p. 950-957.
McSteen P. et als, "A floret by any other name: control of meristem identity in maize", *Trends in Plant Science* 5 (2000) p. 61-66.
Nour A. A. et als, "Chemical composition of baobab fruit (Adansonia digitata L.)", *Tropical Science 22 (*1980) p. 383-388.
Œuvres complètes de Philippe Aureolus Theophraste Bombast de Hohenheim, dit Paracelse, vol. 2, Bibliothèque Chacornac,(1914) p. 192.
Parkouda C. et al, "Biochemical changes associated with the fermentation of baobab seeds in Maari: An alkaline fermented seeds condiment from western Africa", *Journal of Ethnic Foods* 2 (2015) p. 58-63. Cf F.
Parkouda C., et als, "The microbiology of alkaline-fermentation of indigenous seeds used as food condiments in Africa and Asia", *Critical Reviews in Microbiology* 35 *(*2009) p. 139-156.
Parsa A., "Medicinal plants and drugs of plant origin in Iran", *Qualitas Plantarum etMateriae Vegetabiles 5* (1959) p. 375- 394.
Patrut Adrian et als, "Age and architecture of the largest African Baobabs from Mayotte, France", DRC Sustainable Future*: Journal of Environment, Agriculture, and Energy* 1 (2020) p. 33-47 (DOI 10.37281/DRCSF/1.1.5).
Pearson Alice, "Baobab powder. Its multiple benefits", *Myprotein* (2017) p. 15.
Perez Juia, "Baobab, the pharmacist's tree", Darwin Nutrition 8/12 (2022) p. 1-6.
Revanka Sonjay G.r, "Presentation of fungal infections", *The MERCK Manual* 04 (2021) p. 1-3.
Ray Marie-Céline, "10 plantes diurétiques", La Nutrition. Bon à manger, bon à savoir 19/11 (2020) 1-2.
Salih N. et al, "Phenolics and fatty acids compositions of vitex and baobab seeds used as coffee substitutes in Nuba Mountains, Sudan", *Agriculture And Biology Journal Of North America* 6 (2015) p. 90-93.
Sanogo D. et als, "Evaluation of fruit production of natural stands of Baobab (Adansonia digitata L.) in two climatic zones in Senegal", *Journal of Applied Biosciences* 85 (2015).
Sharma B. K. et als, "Adansonia digitata L. (Malvaceae) a threatened tree species of medicinal impor tance", *Medicinal Plants - International Journal of Phytomedicines and Related Industries* / (2015) p. 173.
Singh S. et als, "Medicinal uses of adansonia digitata l.: an endangered tree species", *Journal of Pharmaceutical and Scientific Innovation* 2 (2013) pp. 14-16.
Soloviev P. et als, "Variabilité des caractères physico-chimiques des fruits de trois espèces ligneuses de cueillette récoltés au Sénégal: Adansonia digitata , Balanites aegyptiaca et Tamarindus indica", *Fruits* 59 (2004,) p. 109-119.

Suliman M. B. et als, "Chemical Composition and Antibacterial Activity of Crude Extracts from Sudanese Medicinal Plant Adansonia digitata L", *Chemistry of Advanced Materials 2* (2017) p. 2

Venter S. M. et als, "Baobab (Adansonia digitata L.) fruit production in communal and conservation land- use types in Southern Africa", *Forest Ecology and Management* 261 (2011) p. 630-639.

Von Linné Carl, Hortus Upsaliensis, exhibens plantas exoticas, Laurentii Salvii (1748) p. 236.

Weng C.-J. et al, "Chemopreventive effects of dietary phytochemicals against cancer invasion and metastasis: Phenolic acids, monophenol, polyphenol, and their derivatives", *Cancer Treatment Reviews* 38 (2012) p. 76-87.

Wickens G. E." The baobab: Africa's upside-down tree", *Kew Bulletin* 37 (1982) p. 173-209.

Yusha'u M. et als, "Antibacterial activity of Adansonia digitata stem bark extracts on some clinical bacterial isolates", *International Journal of Biomedical and Health Sciences 6* (2010) p. 129-135.

Zhigila D. A. et als, "A. Numericaò Taxinomy on Varieties of Adansonia Digitata L", *Annals. Food Science and Technology* 16 (2015) p. 157-160.

6.3 Sittography

"Cancer: the different types of treatment", consulted on 18/06/2023 (https://www.roche.fr/fr/patients/info-patients-cancer/traitement-cancer/traitements- cancer.html) 1-3.

"Conseils santé. Les plantes qui luttent contre les cancers", MeSoigner.fr, Accessed 18/06 (2023) 1-2 (https://www.mesoigner.fr/conseils/590-les-plantes-qui- luttent-contre-les-cancers).

Decrouy Antoine, "Composition of a flower - the different parts of a flower", Projet Ecolo 12/05(2023) 1-3 , Accessed 25/06/2023 (https://www.projetecolo.com/composition-d-une-fleur-les-differentes-parties-d-une- fleur-192.html).

"Glucose", *SCF*, consulted on 26/09/2023 (https://new.societechimiquedefrance.fr/produits/glucose/) p. 1-3.

Joan V. et al, "Amenorrhea" , The MSD Handbook (MD, University of Virginia Health System; Medical Review Jan. 2023), Accessed 18/06 /2023 (https://www.msdmanuals.com/fr/professional/gyn)

"La feuille, description globale", Les Jardins du Gué 27/12 (2010), consulted on 25/06/2023 (https://www.jardinsdugue.eu/la-feuille-description-globale/)

"The baobab in Africa, more than a symbol, a resource: the tree of a thousand uses", *Futura* , consulted on 17/04/2024 (https://www.futura-sciences.com/planete/dossiers/botanique-baobab-arbre-

pharmacist-tree-life-666/page/6/) p. 1-8.
"The parts of a plant", Parlons Sciences 26/01 (2023) 1-3, consulted on 08/03/. 2024(https://parlonssciences.ca/ressources-pedagogiques/documents-information/parts-of-a-plant).
"Plants with properties: febrifuge", Génial Végétal, Accessed on 26/06/2023 (https://www.genialvegetal.net/+-Plantes-propriete-febrifuge-+) p. 1-3.

6.4 Oral sources

AGOSSOU Nounagnon Marcel, lay exorcist in Cotonou AHLEGNAN Émile, traditional doctor in Calavi.
AHOUANGAN Koffi Lucien, traditional doctor in Banamè-Awolokpodji
AKABASSI Benjamin, traditional doctor in Za-Kpota Centre
ALLINHLENON Sylvain, traditional doctor, specialising in fractures and dislocations in Tindji.
ATTINHOUHOU Thomas, traditional doctor in Za-Kpota Centre
AWONON Bienvenu, traditional doctor at Za-Kpota Centre
AWONON Pierre, traditional doctor at Za-Kpota Centre
Daa Bokonon Segan, traditional doctor, diviner, priest of Fa (Bokonon) in Affossogba
Daa Yanon: traditional healer and diviner priest of Fa (Bokonon) in Tindji GOGBE Elie, traditional doctor, specialist in mental illnesses in Davègo. HOUNNON GAHOU Miwakponhami, priest of the Vodun Thron and traditional doctor in Za-Kpota Centre.
HOUNON Pascal, traditional doctor in Za-Kpota centre
KPOHAZOUNDE Alain, Pastor of Celestial Christianity in Agondokpé
KOUDJE Didier, traditional doctor in Za-Kpota-Centre
KOUDJÈ Thon Jérôme, traditional doctor in Za-Kpota Centre
KOUDJÈ Toussaint, traditional doctor in Za-Kpota.
KPONHINTO Gérard, traditional doctor in Za-Kpota Centre LANGBEGNON Hervé, traditional doctor in Bohicon. SONON Pascal, Evangelist of celestial Christianity in Za-Kékéré

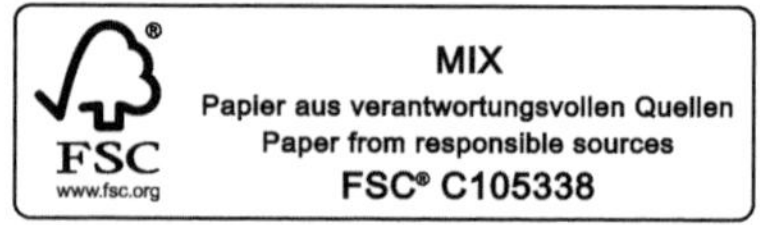

Printed by Books on Demand GmbH, Norderstedt / Germany